T0281471

Updates in Surgery

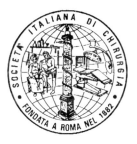

Vittorio Quagliuolo • Alessandro Gronchi
Editors

Current Treatment of Retroperitoneal Sarcomas

A Joint Effort with the
Italian Society of Surgical Oncology

In collaboration with
Ferdinando C.M. Cananzi and Marco Fiore

Foreword by
Marco Montorsi

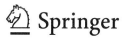 Springer

Editors
Vittorio Quagliuolo
Surgical Oncology Unit
Department of Surgery
Humanitas Clinical and Research
Center
Rozzano, Milan, Italy

Alessandro Gronchi
Sarcoma Service
Department of Surgery
Fondazione IRCCS Istituto Nazionale
dei Tumori
Milan, Italy

The publication and the distribution of this volume have been supported by the Italian Society of Surgery

ISSN 2280-9848   ISSN 2281-0854 (electronic)
Updates in Surgery
ISBN 978-88-470-3979-7   ISBN 978-88-470-3980-3 (eBook)

DOI 10.1007/978-88-470-3980-3

Library of Congress Control Number: 2018948738

Cover design: eStudio Calamar S.L.
External publishing product development: Scienzaperta, Novate Milanese (Milan), Italy
Typesetting: Graphostudio, Milan, Italy

This Springer imprint is published by Springer Nature
The registered company is Springer-Verlag Italia S.r.l.
The registered company address is Via Decembrio 28, I-20137 Milan

Foreword

In 1994 the Italian Society of Surgery inaugurated the series of Biennial Reports aiming at addressing the most current and controversial topics in surgery every year. One of the first two reports dealt with retroperitoneal tumors and was edited by Prof. Davide D'Amico.

After more than twenty years the Society's Executive Board has felt the need to fine-tune the theme of retroperitoneal neoplasias focusing on the most frequent and better studied form, namely sarcomas.

All aspects of this complex disease have considerably evolved in recent years, enriched by new notions in both histological and molecular characterization, as well as in imaging, diagnostic pathways and surgical treatment, increasingly integrated into a multidisciplinary approach which is now essential.

The Editors are two of the most prestigious and competent Italian surgeons, with vast experience on the subject and working in dedicated Institutions with high volumes of oncological activity.

The different aspects of this important disease have been assigned to the most scientifically and clinically active Italian groups to ensure up-to-date and high level cultural development.

The work ends with an interesting chapter that describes the path towards international collaboration of this group of experts to guarantee ever greater integration and exchange of experiences.

I am sure that the monograph of Vittorio Quagliuolo and Alessandro Gronchi will be one of the most appreciated and consulted by the whole surgical community.

Milan, September 2018
Marco Montorsi
President, Italian Society of Surgery

Preface

Retroperitoneal sarcomas (RPS) are rare diseases accounting for 0.15% of all malignant tumors in the adult. Their treatment represents an extraordinary challenge in particular for the surgeon.

Although other modalities may play a role in the management of RPS, surgery remains the cornerstone of therapy. The last 10 years have seen a major change in the surgical approach, with a substantial impact on disease control and cure.

RPS referral centers with dedicated specialists and multidisciplinary tumor boards have become critical to improve disease-specific outcomes as compared with community/general hospitals without this expertise.

National and international collaboration has grown significantly and has clearly proven to be instrumental for conducting research and advancing the knowledge of this rare disease.

In this monograph, we have made an effort to summarize the most recent advances in RPS management: from diagnosis to the management of particular histological subtypes, from neoadjuvant therapies to extended multivisceral resections, with an eye to molecular biology and future perspectives.

Current state-of-the-art knowledge about the various aspects of this complex disease is discussed, covering epidemiology, pathology, genetics, molecular biology, immunology, diagnostics, medical oncology, radiotherapy, prognosis prediction and – of course – surgical management of the different histological subtypes.

The need to adopt a multidisciplinary approach and to regionalize RPS care in few referral centers across the country is often emphasized and is going to be the next challenge to face in the coming years, in order to further improve the prognosis of these patients while awaiting the development of new effective therapies.

We wish to thank the President and the Board of the Italian Society of Surgery for giving us the opportunity and the task of editing this monograph.

Special thanks also to all the contributors to this volume for spending their time to present the many complex aspects of this challenging disease.

A particular thanks to the Italian Society of Surgical Oncology for the active collaboration which has been critical for the preparation of this volume.

Milan, September 2018   Vittorio Quagliuolo
                                                           Alessandro Gronchi

Contents

All web addresses have been checked and were correct at time of printing.

Contributors

Luca Balzarini Department of Radiology, Humanitas Clinical and Research Center, Rozzano

Massimo Barberis Department of Pathology, European Institute of Oncology, Milan, Italy

Alexia F. Bertuzzi Department of Medical Oncology and Hematology, Humanitas Clinical and Research Center, Rozzano, Milan, Italy

Antonella Boglione Department of Oncology, Humanitas Gradenigo Hospital, Turin, Italy

Elena Monica Borroni Department of Biotechnology and Translational Medicine, University of Milan, Italy

Dario Callegaro Sarcoma Service, Department of Surgery, Fondazione IRCCS Istituto Nazionale dei Tumori, Milan, Italy

Ferdinando C.M. Cananzi Department of Biomedical Sciences, Humanitas University, Pieve Emanuele, Milan, and Surgical Oncology Unit, Department of Surgery, Humanitas Clinical and Research Center, Rozzano, Milan, Italy

Umberto Cariboni Department of Thoracic Surgery, Humanitas Clinical and Research Center, Rozzano, Milan, Italy

Maurizio Chiriva-Internati Department of Lymphoma and Myeloma and Department of Gastroenterology, Hepatology and Nutrition, Division of Internal Medicine, The University of Texas MD Anderson Cancer Center, Houston, Texas, USA

Matteo M. Cimino Department of Hepatobiliary and General Surgery, Humanitas Clinical and Research Center, Rozzano, Milan, Italy

Piergiuseppe Colombo Department of Pathology, Humanitas Clinical and Research Center, Rozzano, Milan, Italy

Alessandro Comandone Department of Oncology, Humanitas Gradenigo Hospital, Turin, Italy

Antonino De Paoli Radiation Oncology Department, IRCCS CRO-Aviano, National Cancer Institute, Aviano, Pordenone, Italy

Angelo Paolo Dei Tos University of Padua School of Medicine, Padua, Italy, and Department of Pathology, Azienda ULSS2 Marca Trevigiana, Treviso, Italy

Marco Fiore Sarcoma Service, Department of Surgery, Fondazione IRCCS Istituto Nazionale dei Tumori, Milan, Italy

Jacopo Galvanin Surgical Oncology Unit, Department of Surgery, Humanitas Clinical and Research Center, Rozzano, Milan, Italy

Nicolò Gennaro Training School in Radiology, Humanitas University, Pieve Emanuele, Milan, Italy

Giovanni Grignani Department of Medical Oncology, Candiolo Cancer Institute - FPO IRCCS, Candiolo, Turin, Italy

Fabio Grizzi Department of Immunology and Inflammation, Humanitas Clinical and Research Center, Rozzano, Milan, Italy

Alessandro Gronchi Sarcoma Service, Department of Surgery, Fondazione IRCCS Istituto Nazionale dei Tumori, Milan, Italy

Teresa Mele Department of Oncology, Humanitas Gradenigo Hospital, Turin, Italy

Carlo Morosi Department of Radiology, Fondazione IRCCS Istituto Nazionale dei Tumori, Milan, Italy

Andrea Napolitano Medical Oncology Unit, Campus Bio-Medico University Hospital, Rome, Italy

Federico Navarria Radiation Oncology Department, IRCCS CRO-Aviano, National Cancer Institute, Aviano, Pordenone, Italy

Piera Navarria Radiotherapy and Radiosurgery Department, Humanitas Clinical and Research Center, Rozzano, Milan, Italy

Elisa Palazzari Radiation Oncology Department, IRCCS CRO-Aviano, National Cancer Institute, Aviano, Pordenone, Italy

Elisabetta Pennacchioli Soft Tissue Sarcoma and Rare Tumors Surgical Division, European Institute of Oncology, Milan, Italy

Dorina Qehajaj Department of Immunology and Inflammation, Humanitas Clinical and Research Center, Rozzano, Milan, Italy

Vittorio Quagliuolo Surgical Oncology Unit, Department of Surgery, Humanitas Clinical and Research Center, Rozzano, Milan, Italy

Stefano Radaelli Sarcoma Service, Department of Surgery, Fondazione IRCCS Istituto Nazionale dei Tumori, Milan, Italy

Marco Rastrelli Surgical Oncology Unit, Veneto Institute of Oncology IOV - IRCCS, Padua, Italy

Stefania Rizzo, Department of Radiology, European Institute of Oncology, Milan, Italy

Carlo Riccardo Rossi Surgical Oncology Unit, Veneto Institute of Oncology IOV - IRCCS, and Department of Surgery, Oncology and Gastroenterology, University of Padua, Padua, Italy

Laura Ruspi Surgical Oncology Unit, Department of Surgery, Humanitas Clinical and Research Center, Rozzano, Milan, Italy

Sergio Sandrucci Sarcoma and Rare Visceral Cancers Unit, Città della Salute e della Scienza, University of Turin, Turin, Italy

Roberta Sanfilippo Adult Mesenchymal Tumors and Rare Cancers Medical Oncology Unit, Fondazione IRCCS Istituto Nazionale dei Tumori, Milan, Italy

Claudia Sangalli Radiation Oncology Department, Fondazione IRCCS Istituto Nazionale dei Tumori, Milan, Italy

Marta Sbaraglia Department of Pathology, Azienda ULSS2 Marca Trevigiana, Treviso, Italy

Sanja Stifter Department of Pathology, School of Medicine, University of Rijeka, Croatia

Guido Torzilli Department of Biomedical Sciences, Humanitas University, Pieve Emanuele, Milan, and Department of Hepatobiliary and General Surgery, Humanitas Clinical and Research Center, Rozzano, Milan, Italy

Saveria Tropea Surgical Oncology Unit, Veneto Institute of Oncology IOV - IRCCS, and Department of Surgery, Oncology and Gastroenterology, University of Padua, Padua, Italy

Sergio Valeri General Surgery Unit, Campus Bio-Medico University Hospital, Rome, Italy

Bruno Vincenzi Medical Oncology Unit, Campus Bio-Medico University Hospital, Rome, Italy

History of Surgery in Retroperitoneal Sarcomas

1

Vittorio Quagliuolo, Laura Ruspi, Ferdinando C.M. Cananzi, and Alessandro Gronchi

1.1 Introduction

Sarcomas represent a heterogeneous group of rare malignant tumors with mesenchymal origin that can virtually occur in any anatomic site and account for less than 1% of malignant tumors [1]. They can encompass more than 70 histological subtypes, so that a large number of combinations of primary site and histology exist, with clinically relevant implications in treatment and prognosis [2]. Sarcomas can be grossly divided into three main kinds: soft tissue sarcoma (STS), visceral sarcoma and bone sarcoma [3].

A German analysis reported 6848 cases of sarcoma diagnosed in that country in 2013; among them, STS was the most frequent (70% in men and 74% in women), followed by gastrointestinal stromal tumors (GIST) (22% in men and 18% in women) and bone sarcoma (9% in men and 8% in women). Concerning STS, Ressing et al. found an age-standardized incidence rate per 100,000 of 7.4 in men and 6.6 in women, which is in line with results in the literature [4].

Among STS, retroperitoneal soft tissue sarcomas (RPS) account for approximately 12–15% with a mean incidence of 2.7 cases per million [5, 6].

The retroperitoneum has a wide potential space; therefore, RPS originating in this anatomic district tend to reach very large sizes before they become symptomatic, being often greater than 20 cm in their major axis at the time of diagnosis [7]. Moreover, differently from primary epithelial solid tumors, RPS usually abuts multiple adjacent organs, encasing or infiltrating them [8, 9]. Considering that viscera, major vascular and nervous structures are included in the retroperitoneal space and that macroscopically complete removal of the

V. Quagliuolo (✉)
Surgical Oncology Unit, Department of Surgery, Humanitas Clinical and Research Center
Rozzano, Milan, Italy
e-mail: vittorio.quagliuolo@cancercenter.humanitas.it

V. Quagliuolo, A. Gronchi (Eds), *Current Treatment of Retroperitoneal Sarcomas*,
Updates in Surgery
DOI: 10.1007/978-88-470-3980-3_1, © Springer-Verlag Italia 2019

tumor is nowadays considered as the best approach in order to improve survival, it is clear that surgery for RPS can be really challenging.

Although both radiotherapy and chemotherapy, administered in neoadjuvant or adjuvant settings, alone or combined, may play a role in the management of RPS, surgery remains the cornerstone of the treatment of resectable RPS [8, 10].

1.2   From Morgagni's First Report to Mid-20th Century

The first report of a large retroperitoneal mass in the western literature occurred in 1761 and it is credited to the Italian anatomist Giovanni Battista Morgagni, who found a large lipomatous tumor in the retroperitoneal space during the autopsy of a 60-year-old female [11]. In the following decades, other single cases and limited series of RPS were published; most of these papers were, however, focused predominantly on the clinical presentation or autoptic findings of these tumors, while data on surgery in these patients were only occasionally reported. At the beginning of the 20th century, Dutton Steele described a total of 61 cases of RPS in his paper "A critical summary of the literature on retroperitoneal sarcoma" [12]. Another literature review by Howard Williams accounted for a total of 84 RPS, considering reports from different continents; interestingly, the percentage of surgically treated patients in this review was only 14% [13]. We had to wait until 1933 for the first single-institution series with a relevant number of patients, when Judd published data on 46 patients diagnosed with RPS treated with surgery; most surgical procedures were only biopsies and complete resection of the tumor was described in only 15 (32%) patients. The author did not specify the mortality rate in his series, but a significant local recurrence rate even in RPS treated with wide complete excision was observed [14].

1.3   1950s – 1980s

In 1954 Pack and Tabah published the results of 120 retroperitoneal tumors treated at the Memorial Sloan Kettering Cancer Center between 1926 and 1951. Complete excision of the tumor was achieved in 21% of cases, with a reported operative mortality of 10.8% considering all of the surgical procedures (i.e., including biopsies, partial resections and complete resections) [15].

In 1960s the rate of surgical resection in RPS started to increase, probably as a consequence of a greater awareness of retroperitoneal tumors and maybe earlier detection [16]: 83% of patients were reported to be surgically treated in a series of 41 patients with malignant retroperitoneal neoplasms by Armstrong in 1965 [17]. In 1967, Braasch and Mon described a lower rate of surgically treated RPS (25/37, 67%) but with a rate of curative resections up to 41% and a postoperative mortality rate of 8% [18].

In the 1970s, available results about patients undergoing surgical resection of RPS reported a 5-year disease-free survival rate ranging from 0% to 21%; however, also considering that computed tomography to ascertain recurrence was not widespread at that time, the actual incidence of recurrence may have been underestimated [19].

In 1973, Kinne examined the 25-year experience at the Memorial Hospital for Cancer and Allied Diseases of New York. Considering 34 RPS among 249 liposarcomas, 11 (32.4%) patients underwent complete resection with/without radiation therapy; 15 (44.1%) had partial resection and radiation therapy while 8 (23.5%) only received a biopsy and radiation therapy. Operative mortality was 11.7%. Average survival in the complete excision group was 7 years (range, 30 months–23 years), with a 5-year survival of 64% in radically treated patients [20].

In 1984, McGrath published results for 47 RPS patients who underwent surgery at the Medical College of Virginia. Complete resection was performed in 38% of patients; in 68% of cases curative surgery required multivisceral resection, with kidney (32%), colon (25%) and adrenal gland (18%) being the most frequently resected organs. The complication rate was up to 32%; no postoperative mortality was observed. A correlation between complications and extent of resection/number of resected organs was not tested or – at least – stated in the paper [21].

1.4   1990s – Today

At the beginning of 1990s, the results of surgery for RPS, even after complete resection, were still poor. This led the authors to call for cooperation between different centers and the establishment of a national registry aiming "to evaluate and track these unusual neoplasms" [22].

The extent of resection and the optimal margin were still far from being defined, and the role of non-surgical therapies had never been formally evaluated.

In 1998, in a large single-institution series of RPS (considering both primary and recurrent tumors), Lewis demonstrated the relevance of complete resection on the outcome of 500 patients treated over a 15-year period. His results showed a significantly longer overall survival (OS) for patients who received complete resection compared with patients who had grossly incomplete resection, with a postoperative mortality rate of 4% [24] (Table 1.1). The importance of resection margin status had already been stressed by Singer in 1995, in a series of 183 patients with both truncal and retroperitoneal sarcoma. At multivariate analysis, both high-grade histology and margins of resection were found to be important independent prognostic factors for survival in RPS [25].

Table 1.1 Historical series reporting on retroperitoneal sarcoma surgery

Author	Period	No. of patients with primary RPS	Complete resection	Morbidity	Mortality	5-year survival in complete resection
Pack and Tabah [15]	1926- 1951	120	21.0%	n.a.	10.8%	n.a.
Kinne et al. [20]	1940- 1965	34	32.4%	n.a.	11,7%	64%
McGrath et al. [21]	1964- 1982	47	38.3%	33%.	0	70%
Cody et al. [19]	1971- 1977	80	66.0%	n.a.	3.7%	45%
Jaques et al. [23]	1982- 1987	63	65.1%	14% major 9% minor	4.0%	74%
Lewis et al. [24]	1982- 1997	278	80.0%	n.a.	4.0%	60%

RPS, retroperitoneal sarcoma; *n.a.*, not available.

In the 2000s, two major European sarcoma groups (Gronchi and colleagues in Italy and Bonvalot and colleagues in France) introduced a new concept of radical resection, by performing a frontline extended surgery with the removal of all adjacent organs in conjunction with the primary tumor, even if not overtly infiltrated (i.e., compartmental resection).

Results from the French Sarcoma Group (a multi-institutional series involving 382 patients) were published in 2009. The group retrospectively reviewed operative reports of patients who underwent surgery for primary RPS showing that extended resection was associated with a 3.29-fold reduced risk of local recurrence compared with patients treated with simple complete resection (p=0.004) [5].

In the same issue of the Journal of Clinical Oncology, Gronchi from the Istituto Nazionale Tumori (INT) in Milan reported results for 288 patients treated with standard resection or extended resection. Similarly to Bonvalot, the Italian group found improved rates of recurrence-free survival (RFS) in patients treated by compartmental resection (5-year recurrence rate, 28%) compared with standard resection (5-year recurrence rate, 48%) [26].

Major criticisms were raised in response to these two studies, especially from American authors, and a debate on the extent of resection arose among the different referral centers for sarcoma surgery [27–29]. It was claimed the study had a high reoperation rate and a probable underestimation of the morbidity rate, the latter partially due to its retrospective nature [28]. Strauss instead focused his criticism on the hypothesis that an improved OS could derive from a selective and liberal approach to resection of some adjacent organs (kidney, psoas muscle, colon) while preserving other adjacent critical structures (major vessels, namely: inferior vena cava, aorta, superior mesenteric artery) [30]. Although critics against compartmental resection argue that organ preservation is less morbid [31], a conservative surgical management seems to be associated with a similar reoperation rate, although a lower morbidity rate has been reported [32].

In more recent years, since the histologic subtype has been reported to be the most important predictive factor of local recurrence and distant metastasis [33, 34], surgery went towards not only an anatomy-guided, but also a tumor biology-oriented approach [35]. Different histologic subtypes show distinct patterns of recurrence (local or distant) and a peculiar likelihood of histopathologic organ invasion; therefore, clinicians should consider this issue when planning treatment for each single patient.

Awareness of the heterogeneity, rarity and complexity of RPS led treating clinicians to appreciate the need for a multidisciplinary approach in referral centers in order to optimize sarcoma treatment (both surgical and non-surgical). Indeed, it is now widely recognized that the expertise of the referral center is crucial and represents one of the most significant factors affecting survival in STS [36, 37]. In 2017, the European CanCer Organization (ECCO) published a statement of essential requirements for quality cancer care in STS in order to establish a high-quality service for sarcoma patients. Surgeons, medical oncologists, radiologists and interventional radiologists, pathologists, radiotherapists and nurses all collaborate in the complex pathway of sarcoma care as a multidisciplinary team [38]. Again, the adequacy of the surgical oncology department had to be assured by a certain volume of procedures per year; high case volume in fact proved to be an independent predictor of favorable outcome in sarcoma surgery [37]. Finally, the centralization of sarcoma care in referral hospitals should make it easier to create a nationwide review and reporting standard [39].

This monograph aims to provide a comprehensive and updated review of the management of RPS, emphasizing the key role of a multidisciplinary and specialized approach. The concepts and pathways of care illustrated in each chapter mainly originate from current scientific evidence but also from the specific expertise of the authors. They should serve as a guide when evaluating and treating patients with RPS while also helping to recognize complex clinical scenarios deserving referral to tertiary care centers.

References

1. Gatta G, van der Zwan JM, Casali PG et al; RARECARE Working Group (2011) Rare cancers are not so rare: the rare cancer burden in Europe. Eur J Cancer 47(17):2493–2511

2. Stiller CA, Trama A, Serraino D et al; RARECARE Working Group (2013) Descriptive epidemiology of sarcomas in Europe: report from the RARECARE project. Eur J Cancer 49(3):684–695
3. Fletcher C, Bridge JA Hogendoorn P, Mertens F (eds) (2013) WHO Classification of tumours of soft tissue and bone, 4th edn. IARC Press, Lyon
4. Ressing M, Wardelmann E, Hohenberger P et al (2018) Strengthening health data on a rare and heterogeneous disease: sarcoma incidence and histological subtypes in Germany. BMC Public Health 18(1):235
5. Bonvalot S, Rivoire M, Castaing M et al (2009) Primary retroperitoneal sarcomas: a multivariate analysis of surgical factors associated with local control. J Clin Oncol 27(1):31–37
6. Messiou C, Moskovic E, Vanel D et al (2017) Primary retroperitoneal soft tissue sarcoma: Imaging appearances, pitfalls and diagnostic algorithm. Eur J Surg Oncol 43(7):1191–1198
7. Chouairy CJ, Abdul-Karim FW, MacLennan GT (2007) Retroperitoneal liposarcoma. J Urol 177(3):1145
8. Bonvalot S, Raut CP, Pollock RE et al (2012) Technical considerations in surgery for retroperitoneal sarcomas: position paper from E-Surge, a master class in sarcoma surgery, and EORTC-STBSG. Ann Surg Oncol 19(9):2981–2991
9. Mussi C, Colombo P, Bertuzzi A et al (2011) Retroperitoneal sarcoma: is it time to change the surgical policy? Ann Surg Oncol 18(8):2136–2142
10. Casali PG, Abecassis N, Bauer S et al (2018) Soft tissue and visceral sarcomas: ESMO-EURACAN Clinical Practice Guidelines for diagnosis, treatment and follow-up. Ann Oncol [Epub ahead of print] doi:10.1093/annonc/mdy096
11. Morgagni GB (1761) De sedibus et causis morborum per anatomen indagatis. Typographia Remondiniana, Venice
12. Steele JD (1900) A critical summary of the literature on retroperitoneal sarcoma. Am J Med Sci 119:311
13. Williams HJ (1903) Primary retroperitoneal sarcoma. Am J Med Sci 126:269–276
14. Judd ES, Larson LM (1933) Retroperitoneal tumors. S Clin North America 12:823
15. Pack GT, Tabah EJ (1954) Primary retroperitoneal tumors: a study of 120 cases. Int Abstr Surg 99(3):209–231
16. Tseng WW, Seo HJ, Pollock RE, Gronchi A (2018) Historical perspectives and future directions in the surgical management of retroperitoneal sarcoma. J Surg Oncol 117(1):7–11
17. Armstrong JR, Cohn I Jr (1965) Primary malignant retroperitoneal tumors. Am J Surg 110(6):937–943
18. Braasch JW, Mon AB (1967) Primary retroperitoneal tumors. Surg Clin North Am 47(3):663–678
19. Cody HS 3rd, Turnbull AD, Fortner JG, Hajdu SI (1981) The continuing challenge of retroperitoneal sarcomas. Cancer 47(9):2147–2152
20. Kinne DW, Chu FC, Huvos AG et al (1973) Treatment of primary and recurrent retroperitoneal liposarcoma. Twenty-five-year experience at Memorial Hospital. Cancer 31(1):53–64
21. McGrath PC, Neifeld JP, Lawrence W Jr et al (1984) Improved survival following complete excision of retroperitoneal sarcomas. Ann Surg 200(2):200–204
22. Storm FK, Mahvi DM (1991) Diagnosis and management of retroperitoneal soft-tissue sarcoma. Ann Surg 214(1):2–10
23. Jaques DP, Coit DG, Hajdu SI, Brennan MF (1990) Management of primary and recurrent soft-tissue sarcoma of the retroperitoneum. Ann Surg 212(1):51–59.
24. Lewis JJ, Leung D, Woodruff JM, Brennan MF (1998) Retroperitoneal soft-tissue sarcoma: analysis of 500 patients treated and followed at a single institution. Ann Surg 228(3):355–365
25. Singer S, Corson JM, Demetri GD et al (1995) Prognostic factors predictive of survival for truncal and retroperitoneal soft-tissue sarcoma. Ann Surg 221(2):185–195

26. Gronchi A, Lo Vullo S, Fiore M et al (2009) Aggressive surgical policies in a retrospectively reviewed single-institution case series of retroperitoneal soft tissue sarcoma patients. J Clin Oncol 27(1):24–30

27. Pisters PW (2009) Resection of some – but not all – clinically uninvolved adjacent viscera as part of surgery for retroperitoneal soft tissue sarcomas. J Clin Oncol 27(1):6–8

28. Raut CP, Swallow CJ (2010) Are radical compartmental resections for retroperitoneal sarcomas justified? Ann Surg Oncol 17(6):1481–1484

29. Gronchi A, Pollock R (2011) Surgery in retroperitoneal soft tissue sarcoma: a call for a consensus between Europe and North America. Ann Surg Oncol 18(8):2107–2110

30. Strauss DC, Hayes AJ, Thomas JM (2011) Retroperitoneal tumours: review of management. Ann R Coll Surg Engl 93(4):275–280

31. Pasquali S, Vohra R, Tsimopoulou I et al (2015) Outcomes following extended surgery for retroperitoneal sarcomas: results from a UK referral centre. Ann Surg Oncol 22(11): 3550–3556

32. Strauss DC, Hayes AJ, Thway K et al (2010) Surgical management of primary retroperitoneal sarcoma. Br J Surg 97(5):698–706

33. Tan MC, Brennan MF, Kuk D et al (2016) Histology-based classification predicts pattern of recurrence and improves risk stratification in primary retroperitoneal sarcoma. Ann Surg 263(3):593–600

34. Callegaro D, Miceli R, Bonvalot S et al (2016) Development and external validation of two nomograms to predict overall survival and occurrence of distant metastases in adults after surgical resection of localised soft-tissue sarcomas of the extremities: a retrospective analysis. Lancet Oncol 17(5):671–680

35. Fairweather M, Gonzalez RJ, Strauss D, Raut CP (2018) Current principles of surgery for retroperitoneal sarcomas. J Surg Oncol 117(1):33–41

36. Venigalla S, Nead KT, Sebro R et al (2018) Association between treatment at high-volume facilities and improved overall survival in soft tissue sarcomas. Int J Radiat Oncol Biol Phys 100(4):1004–1015

37. Sandrucci S, Trama A, Quagliuolo V, Gronchi A (2017) Accreditation for centers of sarcoma surgery. Updates Surg 69(1):1–7

38. Andritsch E, Beishon M, Bielack S et al (2017) ECCO essential requirements for quality cancer care: soft tissue sarcoma in adults and bone sarcoma. A critical review. Crit Rev Oncol Hematol 110:94–105

39. Hoekstra HJ, Haas RLM, Verhoef C et al (2017) Adherence to guidelines for adult (non-GIST) soft tissue sarcoma in the Netherlands: a plea for dedicated sarcoma centers. Ann Surg Oncol 24(11):3279–3288

The Pathology of Retroperitoneal Sarcomas

Marta Sbaraglia, Piergiuseppe Colombo,
and Angelo Paolo Dei Tos

2.1   Introduction

Soft tissue sarcomas are a heterogeneous group of rare malignancies with an annual incidence of approximately 5 per 100,000 individuals and therefore represent less than 1.5% of all human malignancies [1]. They are characterized by destructive growth, recurrence and distant metastases most often to the lungs. Any anatomic site may be affected, although most often sarcomas occur in the deep soft tissue of the extremities. The retroperitoneum is involved as a primary site in about 15–20% of cases. In principle, any sarcoma subtype can arise at this location, but a limited number of lesions exhibit a higher anatomic tropism. The most common histotypes that exhibit a tendency to occur in the retroperitoneum are represented by well-differentiated/dedifferentiated liposarcomas, leiomyosarcomas, solitary fibrous tumors, malignant peripheral nerve sheath tumors and undifferentiated pleomorphic sarcomas [1]. It has to be also underlined, however, that sarcomas represent only one-third of retroperitoneal neoplasms, making the differential diagnoses with non-mesenchymal tumor challenging.

The retroperitoneal location is most often associated with a worse prognosis if compared with the extremities. In fact, at this anatomic location tumors have a tendency to attain larger size, which is associated with a comparatively lesser chance to achieve complete surgical excision.

M. Sbaraglia (✉)
Department of Pathology, Azienda ULSS2 Marca Trevigiana
Treviso, Italy
e-mail: marta.sbaraglia@aulss2.veneto.it

V. Quagliuolo, A. Gronchi (Eds), *Current Treatment of Retroperitoneal Sarcomas*,
Updates in Surgery
DOI: 10.1007/978-88-470-3980-3_2, © Springer-Verlag Italia 2019

2.2   Well-differentiated and Dedifferentiated Liposarcomas

By far the most frequent histotypes in retroperitoneal sarcoma are represented by well-differentiated liposarcoma (WDLPS) and dedifferentiated liposarcoma (DDLPS) [2]. Both are MDM2-driven tumors; however, whereas WDLPS is incapable of systemic spread, DDLPS has not only increased local aggressiveness (which indeed accounts for most of the disease-related mortality) but can also metastasize in approximately 20% of cases. Three subtypes of WDLPS are currently recognized by the 2013 WHO classification of soft tissue tumors: (1) adipocytic (or lipoma-like), (2) sclerosing, and (3) inflammatory [3]. Retroperitoneal WDLPS has a high tendency to recur locally, far higher than when occurring at superficial sites. The currently preferred treatment of WDLPS/DDLPS is surgical resection, which should include adjacent viscera [4]. This strategy is aimed to reduce the risk of local recurrence or at least delay the time to the first local recurrence and hopefully prolong overall survival [5]. As multivisceral resection is associated with higher morbidity (an unnecessary risk when dealing with other pleomorphic sarcomas occurring in the retroperitoneum), accurate recognition of WDLPS/DDLPS is a key step in clinical decision-making. Recently published evidence has shown that application of the French National Federation of Comprehensive Cancer Centers (FNCLLC) grading system may help to stratify DDLPS prognostically [6]. Furthermore, the presence of rhabdomyoblastic differentiation is associated with poorer prognosis [6].

Microscopically, lipoma-like WDLPS is composed of a mature adipocytic proliferation featuring striking variation in cell size and nuclear atypia both in fat cells and in stromal cells (Fig. 2.1a) [2]. Importantly, the number of lipoblasts (uni- or multivacuolated fat cells containing a hyperchromatic, scalloped nucleus) is extremely variable (from many to none). Very rarely, foci of metaplastic bone, scattered rhabdomyoblasts, or areas of smooth muscle differentiation can be observed [3]. Sclerosing WDLPS occurs typically in the retroperitoneum. Microscopically, it is characterized by the presence of scattered bizarre, hyperchromatic stromal cells set in a fibrillary background (Fig. 2.1b). The amount of mature fat is very variable and often the fibrous component can predominate [3]. The inflammatory variant of WDLPS is also most frequently seen in the retroperitoneum and is characterized microscopically by the presence of a dense chronic inflammatory infiltrate [7]. As the adipocytic component can be minimal, the detection of scattered atypical stromal cells represents the key morphologic clue to diagnosis (Fig. 2.1c).

Dedifferentiated liposarcoma is traditionally defined as the abrupt transition from WDLPS to non-lipogenic (most often high-grade) sarcoma (Fig. 2.2a). However, such transition sometimes is not abrupt, can be lipogenic and rarely may feature a "low-grade" appearance. Dedifferentiated areas exhibit a remarkable histologic variability. In addition to undifferentiated pleomorphic

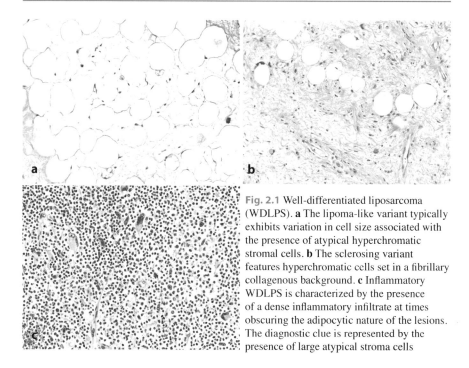

Fig. 2.1 Well-differentiated liposarcoma (WDLPS). **a** The lipoma-like variant typically exhibits variation in cell size associated with the presence of atypical hyperchromatic stromal cells. **b** The sclerosing variant features hyperchromatic cells set in a fibrillary collagenous background. **c** Inflammatory WDLPS is characterized by the presence of a dense inflammatory infiltrate at times obscuring the adipocytic nature of the lesions. The diagnostic clue is represented by the presence of large atypical stroma cells

sarcoma-like morphology, high-grade myxofibrosarcoma-like features are observed. Interestingly, DDLPS may exhibit the presence of fascicles of bland spindle cells with a cellularity somewhat intermediate between well-differentiated liposarcoma sclerosing liposarcoma and usual high-grade areas, termed "low grade dedifferentiation" [3]. Heterologous elements are observed in about 5–10% of cases: most often leiomyosarcomatous, rhabdomyoblastic or osteo/chondrogenic (Fig. 2.2b) [8]. A peculiar morphologic presentation of DDLPS is represented by the presence of whorls of spindle cells somewhat reminiscent of neural or meningothelial structures. The dedifferentiated component may rarely exhibit lipogenic features overlapping morphologically with pleomorphic liposarcoma (i.e., "homologous" dedifferentiation) [9]. Very rarely an intense inflammatory infiltrate is observed to the extent that it may obscure the lipogenic nature of the neoplasm. These cases have been regarded as inflammatory variants of malignant fibrous histiocytoma, although it is now broadly accepted (and genetically demonstrated) that they all represent examples of DDLPS.

As a consequence of amplification occurring in the 12q13-15 chromosome region, overexpression of *MDM2* and *CDK4* is consistently observed in both lipogenic and non-lipogenic components. When dealing with core biopsies of retroperitoneal pleomorphic mesenchymal neoplasm, the demonstration of MDM2 nuclear overexpression strongly supports the diagnosis of DDLPS

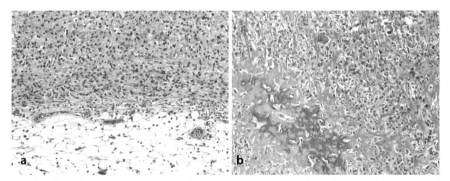

Fig. 2.2 Dedifferentiated liposarcoma (DDLPS). **a** Abrupt transition from well-differentiated liposarcoma (WDLPS) to high-grade non-lipogenic sarcoma is the most frequent morphologic presentation. **b** The presence of heterologous osteosarcomatous differentiation represent a rare but well-recognized finding

[10]. In the case of lipoma-like WDLPS immunostains may at times prove unsatisfactory, making FISH analysis a more consistent diagnostic tool [11].

The differential diagnosis of WDLPS is mainly with benign lipoma which, however, is exceedingly rare in the retroperitoneum. In principle, any lipomatous tumor at this location should be regarded as malignant unless (genetically) proven otherwise [11]. DDLPS needs to be kept separate from other pleomorphic sarcomas that may occur in the retroperitoneum (most often pleomorphic leiomyosarcoma and pleomorphic liposarcoma) as well as from non-sarcomatous lesions such as sarcomatoid carcinoma. Pleomorphic liposarcoma and pleomorphic leiomyosarcoma are ruled out on the basis of the absence of *MDM2* overexpression and/or *MDM2* gene amplification [10]. As mentioned, DDLPS can express myogenic markers generating significant morphologic overlaps with true myogenic neoplasms [8]. Sarcomatoid carcinoma (particularly of renal origin) may also represent at times a major challenge; however, it almost always expresses cytokeratin and/or EMA.

Myxofibrosarcoma-like DDLPS may be mistaken for myxoid liposarcoma. Myxoid liposarcoma, however, arises primarily in the retroperitoneum only exceptionally, never features nuclear pleomorphism and never expresses *MDM2*. *MDM2* overexpression/amplification also differentiates homologous-type DDLPS from pleomorphic liposarcoma [10].

Inflammatory variants of DDLPS need to be differentiated form hematolymphoid malignancies, in particular anaplastic large cell lymphoma (that consistently expresses CD30 and variably stains for ALK) and Castelman's disease. Careful histologic examination most often allows the recognition of scattered atypical cells featuring enlarged hyperchromatic nuclei that are more easily picked-up with *MDM2* immunostaining. In our experience renal angiomyolipoma is at times mistaken for DDLPS. Co-expression of myogenic and melanocytic differentiation markers (HMB45 and/or Melan-A) and *MDM2* negativity allows proper classification in most cases.

2.3   Leiomyosarcoma

Leiomyosarcoma (LMS) represents a malignant mesenchymal neoplasm exhibiting morphologic and immunophenotypic features of smooth muscle differentiation [1]. Leiomyosarcoma occurs predominantly in adult or elderly patients. The retroperitoneal location accounts for approximately 45% of cases and represent a major adverse prognostic factor. At this anatomic site, LMS may arise from the muscular wall of large blood vessels (i.e., inferior vena cava). Retroperitoneal LMS frequently spreads to the lungs and liver with a 5-year overall survival of about 40%.

Microscopically, LMS is composed of fascicles of spindle cells containing blunt-ended nuclei and featuring a distinctive eosinophilic fibrillary cytoplasm (Fig. 2.3a). In high-grade LMS significant pleomorphism is associated with more abundant, often atypical mitotic figures, and variable amounts of necrosis (Fig. 2.3b) [12]. Numerous morphologic variants of LMS exist, such as myxoid, epithelioid, giant cell rich and inflammatory. The morphology is supported by immunohistochemical expression of smooth muscle differentiation markers. Approximately 70–80% of LMS stain for desmin, 60% for h-caldesmon and a vast majority will stain with smooth muscle actin. Genetically, LMS typically shows complex karyotypes with amplification, losses and gains occurring in several chromosomes [13].

The most important differential diagnosis is with leiomyoma which, although it can rarely feature degenerative nuclear atypia, consistently lacks necrosis and

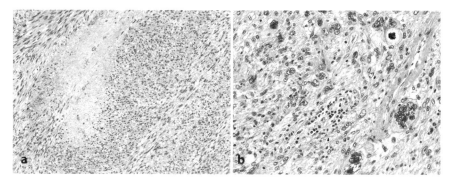

Fig. 2.3 Leiomyosarcoma (LMS). **a** The presence of fascicles of spindle cells containing blunt-ended nuclei and featuring a distinctive eosinophilic fibrillary cytoplasm represents the diagnostic hallmark of LMS. **b** Significant pleomorphism associated with abundant atypical mitoses is observe in high-grade LMS

high mitotic activity [14]. Different criteria apply to male and female patients. In the retroperitoneal smooth muscle neoplasms of females, whenever nuclear atypia is mild to absent, up to 10 mitoses/50 HPF are allowed. When dealing with identical lesions occurring in the retroperitoneum of male patients the application of the above-mentioned diagnostic criteria is not advised [14]. As already mentioned, the differential diagnosis includes DDLPS and is based on the absence of *MDM2* overexpression/amplification [10].

2.4   Solitary Fibrous Tumor

Solitary fibrous tumor (SFT) is a spindle cell neoplasm of adults that in the past has been most often labeled with the now obsolete term "hemangiopericytoma" (HPC) [1]. It is in fact clearly stated in the latest WHO classification that hemangiopericytoma is a term erroneously used to encompass a wide variety (both benign and malignant) of unrelated lesions sharing the presence of an HPC-like vascular network [1]. Pleura, limbs, retroperitoneum, mediastinum, meninges, and pelvis represent the main anatomic locations.

Microscopically, SFT is characterized by a mixed of hypocellular and hypercellular areas composed of monomorphic spindle cell proliferation, organized in a short storiform growth pattern. A distinctive HPC-like vascular network, composed of thin-walled, branching vessels is the diagnostic hallmark (Fig. 2.4a). Dedifferentiated SFT represents the rarest variant and is characterized by transition to high grade pleomorphic morphology [15]. The presence of a variably abundant mature fat component identifies the "fat forming" variant of SFT. Immunohistochemically, SFT typically exhibits positivity for the ubiquitously expressed antigen CD34 (Fig. 2.4b). Much

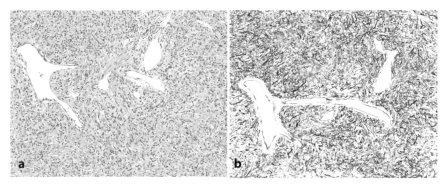

Fig. 2.4 Solitary fibrous tumor (SFT). **a** A monomorphic spindle cell proliferation, organized in a short storiform growth pattern and associated with a hemangiopericytoma-like (HPC-like) vascular network, represents the diagnostic hallmark of SFT. **b** Diffuse CD34 immunopositivity is observed in most cases

greater diagnostic value is attributed to the nuclear expression of *STAT6* [16], which represents the phenotypic consequence of the *NAB2-STAT6* gene fusion [17]. In the retroperitoneum the differential diagnosis of SFT is rather limited and includes those rare examples of DDLPS exhibiting SFT-like features.

Approximately 10% of cases behave aggressively. Metastases are most frequently observed in the lungs, bone and liver. Deeply located lesions appear to behave more aggressively. Malignant behavior seems to be associated with the presence of cytologic atypia, increased cellularity, mitotic activity greater than 4 mitoses/10 HPF, and necrosis [18]; however, their absence does not exclude per se the possibility of an aggressive clinical course.

2.5 Malignant Peripheral Nerve Sheath Tumor

Malignant peripheral nerve sheath tumor (MPNST) represents a spindle cell sarcoma showing morphologic features of nerve sheath differentiation, not necessarily arising from a peripheral nerve [1]. The retroperitoneum, limbs and trunk are among the most commonly affected anatomic sites, followed by the head and neck region. Malignant peripheral nerve sheath tumor generally occurs in adult patients and is regarded as very rare in the pediatric population [19]. The association with neurofibromatosis type 1 (NF-1) is observed in approximately 30–50% of cases [20] and in this scenario the tumor often arises from a pre-existing (plexiform) neurofibroma. The lifetime risk for a NF-1 patient of developing MPNST ranges approximately between 2% and 15%. In NF-1-associated tumors, the peak incidence is earlier than in sporadic forms.

Overall survival at 5 years seems to be affected by clinical presentation, being approximately 50% in sporadic cases, 25% in NF-1 patients and 15% in postirradiation cases. Metastatic spread to the lungs represents the most frequent cause of death. From the therapeutic standpoint complete surgery represents the mainstay. Microscopically, MPNST is composed of a spindle cell proliferation featuring pointed, wavy nuclei. The presence of significant variation in cellularity associated with angiocentric clustering of neoplastic cells is often seen (Fig. 2.5a). Overt pleomorphism represents a rare feature. Palisading represents a relatively rare finding and is actually more often seen in synovial sarcoma and leiomyosarcoma. In approximately 10–15% of cases heterologous differentiation is observed. Such a phenomenon appears to be more common in NF-1 patients. The heterologous component can be osteogenic, chondrogenic, angiosarcomatous, epithelial, but most often is rhabdomyosarcomatous (so-called malignant triton tumor) (Fig. 2.5b) and is associated with a worse prognosis [21].

As mentioned, most examples of MPNST are high-grade, although low-grade MPNST does exist and represents tumor progression occurring in a

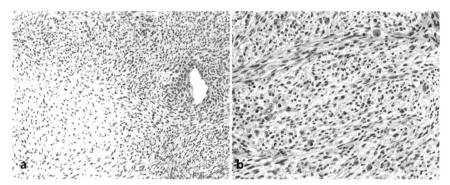

Fig. 2.5 Malignant peripheral nerve sheath tumor (MPNST). **a** Variation and perivascular accentuation of cellularity are typical morphologic features of MPNST. **b** The presence of rhabdomyoblastic heterologous differentiation defines the so-called malignant triton tumor

pre-existing benign neural lesion [22], most often a plexiform neurofibroma in context the of a NF-1 syndrome. The presence of multifocal nuclear atypia and increased cellularity per se does not represent a sufficient criterion of malignancy and a diagnosis of atypical neurofibroma seems to be appropriate in these cases. However, whenever those morphologic features are associated with any mitotic activity, a diagnosis of low-grade MPNST should be rendered [22]. Immunophenotypically, MPNST rarely express S-100 protein, but immunoreactivity is usually limited to a fraction of the neoplastic cell. Glial fibrillary acidic protein (GFAP)-positivity is also observed in less than one-third of cases. Loss of expression of H3K27me3 (determined by PRC2 inactivation via inactivating mutations of either *SUZ12* or *EED1* genes) appears to be fairly specific for MPNST [23]. At the molecular level NF-1 deletions are often observed in both the NF-1 and non-NF-1 groups.

In the retroperitoneum the most important differential diagnosis is represented by cellular schwannoma [24], a mitotically active spindle cell benign neoplasm, featuring a predominant Antoni-A growth pattern. A distinctive hyalinization of the vessel walls represents a key morphologic feature. At variance with MPNST, cellular schwannoma is always well-circumscribed, expresses diffusely S-100 and features a variable amount of EMA-positive perineurial cells at the periphery [24].

Among malignant lesions the differential diagnoses include LMS and monophasic synovial sarcoma. As mentioned, LMS is distinguished by the presence of its distinctive morphology as well as by the expression of smooth muscle markers. Synovial sarcoma is ruled out on the basis of expression of epithelial differentiation markers (EMA and cytokeratin) and also by the presence of the *SYT-SSX* gene fusion. *MDM2* overexpression/amplification allows separating malignant triton tumor from DDLPS with myogenic differentiation [10].

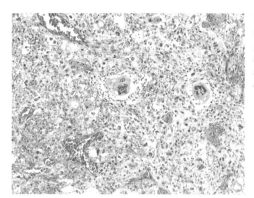

Fig. 2.6 Undifferentiated pleomorphic sarcoma (UPS). The presence of a high grade pleomorphic cell population associated with atypical mitoses and absence of any line of differentiation defines UPS

2.6   Undifferentiated Pleomorphic Sarcoma

The 2013 WHO classification recognizes the existence of an undifferentiated, unclassifiable category of pleomorphic sarcoma [1] and defines it as a group of high-grade sarcomas in which any attempt to disclose their line of differentiation has failed. It has to be underlined that this is a diagnosis of exclusion following thorough sampling and application of ancillary techniques. Most of these cases in the past have contributed to the category malignant fibrous histiocytoma [25]. Currently, undifferentiated pleomorphic sarcoma (UPS) accounts for no more than 10% of sarcomas occurring in adults. The retroperitoneum represents a possible location for UPS wherein rapid growth is most often observed. They typically arise from the muscular structure of the retroperitoneum (i.e., iliopsoas muscle). About 5% of patients exhibit distant metastases to the lungs at presentation. Microscopically, these lesions all share marked pleomorphism. A high number of atypical mitotic figures and abundant necrosis are most often seen (Fig. 2.6). As mentioned, immunohistochemistry does not identify specific lines of differentiation. Before rendering a diagnosis of UPS it is obviously important to exclude the specific sarcoma subtypes featuring pleomorphic morphology (DDLPS and LMS) [10, 12] discussed previously as well as non-mesenchymal mimics such as sarcomatoid carcinoma and metastatic sarcomatoid melanoma.

2.7   Conclusion

In conclusion, sarcomas occurring in the retroperitoneum represent a heterogeneous and challenging group of malignancies. In consideration of the distinctive clinical behaviors, accurate recognition is crucial to allow proper therapeutic strategy.

References

1. Fletcher CD (2014) The evolving classification of soft tissue tumours: an update based on the new 2013 WHO classification. Histopathology 64(1):2–11
2. Dei Tos AP (2014) Liposarcomas: diagnostic pitfalls and new insights. Histopathology 64(1):38–52
3. Evans HL (2007) Atypical lipomatous tumor, its variants, and its combined forms: a study of 61 cases, with a minimum follow-up of 10 years. Am J Surg Pathol 31(1):1–14
4. Gronchi A, Lo Vullo S, Fiore M et al (2009) Aggressive surgical policies in a retrospectively reviewed single-institution case series of retroperitoneal soft tissue sarcoma patients. J Clin Oncol 27(1):24–30
5. Bonvalot S, Rivoire M, Castaing M et al (2009) Primary retroperitoneal sarcomas: a multivariate analysis of surgical factors associated with local control. J Clin Oncol 27(1):31–37
6. Gronchi A, Collini P, Miceli R et al (2015) Myogenic differentiation and histologic grading are major prognostic determinants in retroperitoneal liposarcoma. Am J Surg Pathol 39(3):383–393
7. Kraus MD, Guillou L, Fletcher CDM (1997) Well-differentiated inflammatory liposarcoma: an uncommon and easily overlooked variant of a common sarcoma. Am J Surg Pathol 21(5): 518–527
8. Evans HL, Khurana KK, Kemp BL, Ayala AG (1994) Heterologous elements in the dedifferentiated component of dedifferentiated liposarcoma. Am J Surg Pathol 18(11):1150–1157
9. Mariño-Enríquez A, Fletcher CD, Dal Cin P, Hornick JL (2010) Dedifferentiated liposarcoma with "homologous" lipoblastic (pleomorphic liposarcoma-like) differentiation: clinicopathologic and molecular analysis of a series suggesting revised diagnostic criteria. Am J Surg Pathol 34(8):1122–1131
10. Binh MB, Sastre-Garau X, Guillou L et al (2005) MDM2 and CDK4 immunostainings are useful adjuncts in diagnosing well-differentiated and dedifferentiated liposarcoma subtypes: a comparative analysis of 559 soft tissue neoplasms with genetic data. Am J Surg Pathol 29(10):1340–1347
11. Clay MR, Martinez AP, Weiss SW, Edgar MA (2016) MDM2 and CDK4 immunohistochemistry: should it be used in problematic differentiated lipomatous tumors? A new perspective. Am J Surg Pathol 40(12):1647–1652
12. Oda Y, Miyajima K, Kawaguchi K et al (2001) Pleomorphic leiomyosarcoma: clinicopathologic and immunohistochemical study with special emphasis on its distinction from ordinary leiomyosarcoma and malignant fibrous histiocytoma. Am J Surg Pathol 25(8):1030–1038
13. Dei Tos AP, Maestro R, Doglioni C et al (1996) Tumor suppressor genes and related molecules in leiomyosarcoma. Am J Pathol 148(4):1037–1045
14. Fletcher CD, Kilpatrick SE, Mentzel T (1995) The difficulty in predicting behavior of smooth-muscle tumors in deep soft tissue. Am J Surg Pathol 19(1):116–117
15. Mosquera JM, Fletcher CD (2009) Expanding the spectrum of malignant progression in solitary fibrous tumors: a study of 8 cases with a discrete anaplastic component – is this dedifferentiated SFT? Am J Surg Pathol 33(9):1314–1321
16. Doyle LA, Vivero M, Fletcher CD et al (2014) Nuclear expression of STAT6 distinguishes solitary fibrous tumor from histologic mimics. Mod Pathol 27(3):390–395
17. Chmielecki J, Crago AM, Rosenberg M et al (2013) Whole-exome sequencing identifies a recurrent NAB2-STAT6 fusion in solitary fibrous tumors. Nat Genet 45(2):131–132
18. Demicco EG, Wagner MJ, Maki RG et al (2017) Risk assessment in solitary fibrous tumors: validation and refinement of a risk stratification model. Mod Pathol 30(10):1433–1442
19. Ducatman BS, Scheithauer BW, Piepgras DG et al (1986) Malignant peripheral nerve sheath tumors. A clinicopathologic study of 120 cases. Cancer 57(10): 2006–2021

20. King AA, Debaun MR, Riccardi VM, Gutmann DH (2000) Malignant peripheral nerve sheath tumors in neurofibromatosis 1. Am J Med Genet 93(5): 388–392
21. Brooks JS, Freeman M, Enterline HT (1985) Malignant "triton" tumors. Natural history and immunohistochemistry of nine new cases with literature review. Cancer 55(11): 2543–2549
22. Miettinen MM, Antonescu CR, Fletcher CDM et al (2017) Histopathologic evaluation of atypical neurofibromatous tumors and their transformation into malignant peripheral nerve sheath tumor in patients with neurofibromatosis 1 – a consensus overview. Hum Pathol 67:1–10
23. Schaefer IM, Fletcher CD, Hornick JL (2016) Loss of H3K27 trimethylation distinguishes malignant peripheral nerve sheath tumors from histologic mimics. Mod Pathol 29(1):4–13
24. Woodruff JM, Godwin TA, Erlandson RA et al (1981) Cellular schwannoma: a variety of schwannoma sometimes mistaken for a malignant tumor. Am J Surg Pathol 5(8):733–744
25. Fletcher CD (1992) Pleomorphic malignant fibrous histiocytoma: fact or fiction? A critical reappraisal based on 159 tumors diagnosed as pleomorphic sarcoma. Am J Surg Pathol 16(3):213–228

The Complex Nature of Soft Tissue Sarcomas, Including Retroperitoneal Sarcomas

Fabio Grizzi, Elena Monica Borroni, Dorina Qehajaj, Sanja Stifter, Maurizio Chiriva-Internati, and Ferdinando C.M. Cananzi

3.1 The Complexity of Retroperitoneal Sarcomas

Human cancer remains one of the most complex diseases and, despite the impressive advances that have been made in molecular and cell biology, how cancer cells progress through carcinogenesis and acquire their metastatic ability is still widely debated [1]. Cancer is also recognized as a highly heterogeneous disease. In addition, somatic mutations and epigenetic changes, many of which are specific to the individual neoplasm have been reported [2]. Soft tissue sarcomas are uncommon, but generally aggressive tumors which disproportionately affect children and young adults [3]. These cancers have a high rate of morbidity and mortality, and their overall incidence has been increasing at an estimated rate of 26% over the last 2 decades [3]. It is known that the retroperitoneum can host a large group of benign as well as malignant tumors [4]. Retroperitoneal sarcomas are rare and represent a small group of all sarcomas, approximately 15% [5], with two main histological subtypes named liposarcoma (nearly, 70%) and leiomyosarcoma (15%) [4, 6]. It is now accepted that sarcomas represent a heterogeneous family of tumors: the World Health Organization has defined nearly 50 tumor subtypes; these are named largely according to the tissue they most closely resemble [6]. The characterization of soft-tissue sarcomas has evolved as the information provided by histologic analysis has been integrated with preclinical models, immunohistochemical studies, and high-throughput technologies, including gene expression microarrays [6, 7].

F. Grizzi (✉)
Department of Immunology and Inflammation, Humanitas Clinical and Research Center
Rozzano, Milan, Italy
e-mail: fabio.grizzi@humanitasresearch.it

V. Quagliuolo, A. Gronchi (Eds), *Current Treatment of Retroperitoneal Sarcomas*,
Updates in Surgery
DOI: 10.1007/978-88-470-3980-3_3, © Springer-Verlag Italia 2019

3.2   The Complexity of Sarcomagenesis

Human carcinogenesis is one of the most complex phenomena in biology. Soft tissue sarcomas can be described as non-linear dynamic systems that are discontinuous in space and time, but advance through qualitatively different "states" (Fig. 3.1a). A dynamic system depends on a set of different states or possible configuration patterns, and a number of "transitions" from one state to another during a certain interval of time.

The parameter time depends on a large number of variables that are interconnected in a multitude of ways, thus making it extremely difficult to predict the exact time interval between two successive states [8]. The continuous generation of "unstable" states during the course of carcinogenesis has led to every sort of reorganization of different entities due to a change in the parameters on which they depend being physically defined as a "bifurcation" [8, 9], whereas the term "catastrophe" describes a sudden change that occurs as a reaction of the system to a variation in external conditions [10]. In medical sciences, the term bifurcation has mainly been associated to a genomic mutation in a cell that drastically changes its behavior from normal to malignant [11, 10]. Gérard and Goldbeter suggested that whether investigated by means of "bifurcation diagrams", a detailed computational model for the cyclin-dependent kinases network shows how the balance between "quiescence" and "proliferation" is not only affected by "activators" and "inhibitors" of cell cycle progression, but also by growth factors and other external variables, including the extracellular matrix and cell contact inhibition [9].

Today, it is known that genetic aberrations play a pivotal role in many soft-tissue tumors and help identify tumors that were previously difficult to classify, particularly pleomorphic soft-tissue sarcomas [12]. These genetic aberrations have been categorized as hereditary or acquired [13–17]. It has also been reported that specific translocations resulting in new fusion genes characterize the sarcomagenesis [18]. Recently, Drummond et al. reported a transdifferentiation program apparent in rhabdomyosarcomas arising through cell fate reprogramming from single oncogene activation in endothelial cell precursors [19, 20]. It is now clear that integrating genetic information with histopathology features can facilitate the diagnosis, confirm relationships between morphologic subtypes, and predict the complex behavior of specific sarcomas [3, 21, 22]. Heterogeneity is observed at the genetic, proteomic, morphological, and environmental levels [23–25]. It is recognized that this genetic and phenotypical variability determines the self-progressive growth, invasiveness and metastatic potential of neoplastic disease and its response or resistance to therapy [10]. Gene-array and proteomic techniques have been not only introduced to identify specific characteristics of each sub-type, but also new potential therapeutic strategies. Additionally, the "retroperitoneum" is a complex anatomical environment comprising fascial layers, spaces, and inter-

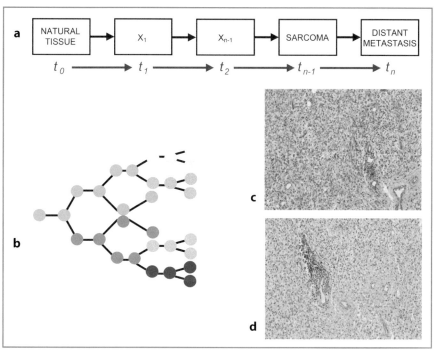

Fig. 3.1 **a** Retroperitoneal sarcomas may be depicted as dynamic systems that are discontinuous in space and time, but advance through qualitatively different "states". A dynamic system depends on a set of different states (x) or possible configuration patterns, and a number of "transitions" from one state to another during a certain interval of time. The parameter time (t) depends on a large number of variables that are interconnected in a multitude of ways, thus making it extremely difficult to predict the exact time interval between two successive states. **b** Sarcomas are highly heterogeneous. Heterogeneity is observed at the genetic, proteomic, morphological (i.e., high number of cell sub-types and distribution patterns), and environmental levels. It is now recognized that this genetic and phenotypical variability determines the self-progressive growth, invasiveness and metastatic potential of neoplastic disease and its response or resistance to therapy. Heterogeneity is essentially a statistical property of cellular populations. A range of cellular behaviors can be estimated from observations of a small number of cells over long times, or a large number of cells at a small number of times. It is known that malignant transformation of cells is associated with down-regulation of HLA class I antigen processing and presenting machinery (APM) components in most of the tumors, including soft tissue sarcomas. These defects are clinically relevant, since they are frequently associated with the clinical course of the disease. Image **c** shows the heterogeneous expression of β2-microglobulin while image **d** shows the complete absence of tapasin in the sarcomatoid component. The protein is only detectable in infiltrating inflammatory cells (objective magnification, 10×).

fascial planes [26]. Several studies have demonstrated that high retroperitoneal visceral fat content increases retroperitoneal soft-tissue sarcoma local recurrence and patients' mortality. Most retroperitoneal soft tissue sarcomas initiate and recur within visceral fat. Loewenstein et al. reported that visceral fat directly interacts with retroperitoneal sarcoma cells by secreting specific adipokines into the tumor microenvironment, thus increasing retroperitoneal soft-tissue sarcoma tumor cell proliferation and invasiveness [27]. Fat-induced soft-tissue sarcoma molecular deregulations should be further investigated to identify new potential prognostic and therapeutic targets.

3.3   The Multi-scale Causality of Retroperitoneal Sarcomas

It is known that the decisive step in carcinogenesis is the result of an irreversible qualitative change in one or more of the genetic characteristics of cancer cells. Although this modification governs the transformation of natural human cells into malignant cancer cells, it may or may not lead to visible changes in their cytological or histological structures [1, 10, 28]. This can be mainly explained using the concept of "emergence", which defines a human being as a complex system consisting of different anatomical entities that are interconnected at many organizational levels, have various degrees of complexity, and are governed by specific laws that only operate at a particular level [28, 1]. Observed processes and patterns can often be conceptualized as macro-scale manifestations of micro-scale processes. Cancers, including sarcoma, are determined by a number of processes and controls operating over much broader scales, and by factors such as structural or functional controls that may operate at scales ranging from molecular to environmental. The results of several lines of research indicate that neoplastic cells share a common set of "acquired capabilities" that operate and are controlled at different spatial and temporal scales, including their abilities: *a)* to generate their own mitogenic signal; *b)* to resist exogenous growth-inhibitory signals; *c)* to evade apoptosis, and senescence; *d)* to proliferate without limit; *e)* to acquire vasculature (i.e. to undergo angiogenesis), and *f)* to invade and metastasize distant organs.

Aside these shared behavioral characteristics each cancer cell is a self-governing entity, which has the capability to progress independently by other surrounding cells.

The Ki-67 protein is strongly associated with cell proliferation, and the Ki-67 labeling index is thus a useful indicator of histological grade for predicting the behavior of soft tissue sarcomas [29].

It is known that blood vessels in tumors are composed of phenotypically different endothelial cells and various amounts of supportive mural cells including pericytes and vascular smooth muscle cells [30]. In 1999, Tomlinson et al. reported that the pattern of angiogenesis is different between sarcomas and carcinomas [31]. Their study showed that the capillaries in carcinomas are clustered within the tumor stroma and that the microvessel density (MVD) can be used as a prognostic factor. Conversely, MVD in sarcomas was shown to have a more homogeneous appearance. A more recent study confirmed this pattern of angiogenesis showing that hot-spots of angiogenesis were diffuse in high-grade soft-tissue tumors and only present in 33% of the investigated specimens [32]. The therapeutic efficacy of anti-angiogenic therapy has been evaluated in several sarcoma clinical trials.

Several investigators have investigated the importance or prognostic relevance of infiltrating immune and inflammatory cells in sarcomas. D'Angelo et al. reported a high prevalence of tumor-infiltrating lymphocytes in soft tissue sarcoma [33]. Interestingly, infiltration of CD8[+] lymphocytes in Ewing sarcoma correlated with improved survival [34]. CD20[+] lymphocytes have been associated with improved survival in a study on soft tissue sarcoma [35]. In 2009 Tseng et al. have highlighted that the presence of CD4[+] T and CD20[+]-lymphocytes in clusters and scattered CD8[+] T-lymphocytes suggest that the naturally occurring immune response in inflammatory, well-differentiated liposarcoma is adaptive and potentially driven by one or more tumor antigens [36]. It is known that malignant transformation of cells is associated with down-regulation of human leukocyte antigen (HLA) class I antigen processing and presenting machinery (APM) components in most of the tumors [37], including soft tissue sarcomas (Fig. 3.1c,d) [38, 39]. These defects are clinically relevant, since they are frequently associated with the clinical course of the disease. Several escape mechanisms have been identified and characterized [40]. Among them, defects in the HLA class I expression and/or function in tumor cells have been extensively investigated because of their potential role in the escape of tumor cells from T cell identification [41, 42]. In humans, CD8[+] T-lymphocytes play an important role in controlling pathogens-infections and malignant cell growth [43, 44]. It has been ascertained that CD8[+] T-lymphocytes recognize cell surface-bound complexes generated by the loading of β2-macroglobulin-associated HLA (β2m-associated HLA) class I heavy chains (HC) with antigen-derived peptides fragments. The generation of these complexes and their transport to the cell membrane depend on well-balanced interactions among the APM molecules. The peptides generated mostly from endogenous proteins by proteasome are transported by a dedicated peptide transporter (TAP, transporter associated with antigen processing), which consists of two sub-units (TAP1 and TAP2), to the lumen of the endoplasmic reticulum (ER)-membrane, where they are loaded on the newly synthesized β2m-associated HLA class I HC with the assistance of the chaperones calnexin, calreticulin, endoplasmic reticulum protein 57 (ERp57), and tapasin. The resulting trimolecular complex subsequently reaches the cell membrane presenting the peptides to CD8[+] T lymphocytes [45–57]. Defects of HLA class I and APM molecules have been shown to be associated with the malignant transformation of cells, although with different frequency in various types of cancers [44, 46, 54, 58–77]. Moreover, they have a negative effect on the clinical progression of the neoplastic disease as well as the outcome of CD8[+] T-lymphocytes-based immunotherapy. Although the critical roles played by HLA class I and APM components in the interactions between malignant cells and immune cells is well established, limited data are available today on their expression in soft tissue sarcoma [39]. Although surgery involving resection of the tumor and involved adjacent structures remains the standard of care for patients with localized retroperitoneal sarcomas [78], immunotherapy has been under development as a novel therapeutic strategy [21, 79–81]. Cancer testis antigens are considered promising immunotherapy targets because of their limited expression in normal tissue [82, 83]. Several investigators have demonstrated a frequent expression of NY-ESO-1 in synovial sarcoma and myxoid/round cell liposarcoma [84]. PRAME was also highly expressed in myxoid/round cell liposarcoma. PRAME and NY-ESO-1 expression was also investigated in histological subtypes of liposarcomas [85]. The authors found that both PRAME and NY-ESO-1 were expressed in most of myxoid/round cell liposarcoma and their expression levels were higher in myxoid/round cell liposarcoma than other liposarcoma types [85]. High expression of PRAME or NY-ESO-1 was correlated with larger tumor size, presence of necrosis, a more than 5% of round cell component, higher histological grade, higher clinical stage and worse prognosis. According to these findings, Iura et al. concluded that PRAME and NY-ESO-1 could be not only useful prognostic markers but also immunotherapeutic targets for myxoid/round cell liposarcoma [85]. The same authors also reported that the immunotherapy targeting MAGEA4 or NY-ESO-1 can be an ancillary therapy in different sarcoma types including, synovial sarcomas, myxoid liposarcomas, osteosarcomas, angiosarcomas, malignant peripheral nerve sheath tumors, and chondrosarcomas [86].

Recently, our understanding of subtype-specific cancer biology has revealed distinct molecular alterations responsible for tumor initiation and progression. These findings have motivated the development of targeted therapies that are being evaluated in subtype-specific or biomarker-driven clinical trials [87, 88]. Although a subset of sarcomas appears inflamed and responsive to immune checkpoint blockade with programmed death 1 (PD-1) targeted agents, novel immunotherapies and combinations likely will be needed for most subtypes. Machado et al. have recently reported that PD-L1 expression was not significantly related to prognosis [89]. Boxberg et al. examined PD-L1 protein and *CD274/ PD-L1* gene copy number variations in 128 primary resected, therapy-naive high-grade sarcomas using immunohistochemistry and fluorescence-in-situ hybridization [90]. Their findings represent novel insights into the immune landscape of soft tissue sarcomas, in particular undifferentiated pleomorphic sarcomas and strengthen the rationale for immunotherapy, including targeting the PD-1/PD-L1 axis in these tumors. However, a recent meta-analysis indicated that high PD-L1 expression is likely to be a negative factor for patients with sarcomas and that it predicts worse survival outcomes [91]. These controversial findings might be partially due to the high heterogeneity of soft tissue sarcomas.

3.4   Concluding Remarks

Despite the rapid advances that have been made in the fields of molecular and cellular biology, there is no doubt that human cancers, including sarcomas, remain very complex disease: it can be hypothesized that each sarcoma type and sub-type are unique, and that the spectrum of biological changes determining these neoplasms is infinitely variable.

Sarcomagenesis may be considered as a non-linear dynamic process that depends on a large number of variables and is regulated at multiple spatial and temporal scales. It is a process, whose behavior does not follow clearly predictable and repeatable pathways. Non-linear systems are characterized by three main properties: a) they do not react proportionally to the magnitude of their inputs; b) they depend on their initial conditions. Small changes in the initial conditions may generate very different end points, and c) their behavior is not deterministic. These characteristics are frequently shown by the fact that it is common to see differences in the progression or therapeutic response of the same tumor type, and the fact that cancer morphology does not always reveal an underlying biology.

The above reflections have led us to think that:

a) Retroperitoneal sarcomas are highly complex and heterogeneous diseases in time and in space.

b) Considering retroperitoneal sarcoma as a robust system would provide us with a framework for future research strategies, and future cancer therapies may be judged on their ability to help control the robustness of tumors.

c) Modeling the growth and development of retroperitoneal sarcomas using mathematics and biological data may be a burgeoning area of cancer research. Mathematical methods and their derivatives have proved to be possible and practical in oncology, but the current models are often simplifications that ignore vast amounts of knowledge.

Analyzing retroperitoneal sarcoma as a dynamically complex system will probably reveal more about its behavioral characteristics. This way of thinking may further help to clarify concepts, interpret new and old experimental data, indicate alternative experiments and categorize the acquired knowledge on the basis of the similitude and/or shared behaviors of very different tumors. Additionally, analysis of the initiation and progression of mesenchymal cancer cells from natural cells and the heterogeneity of a retroperitoneal sarcoma population raises two intriguing questions: a) what are the properties shared by mesenchymal cancer and natural cells? and b) to what extent are these properties shared? Both natural and mesenchymal tumoral cells are networks of sub-cellular anatomical entities organized in such a way as to perform all of the complex functions necessary to guarantee the cell's existence.

It is encouraging that surgeons, clinicians, biologists and mathematicians continue to contribute together towards a common quantitative understanding of retroperitoneal sarcomas complexity.

References

1. Grizzi F, Di Ieva A, Russo C et al (2006) Cancer initiation and progression: an unsimplifiable complexity. Theor Biol Med Model 3:37
2. Widschwendter M, Jones A, Evans I et al; FORECEE (4C) Consortium (2018) Epigenome-based cancer risk prediction: rationale, opportunities and challenges. Nat Rev Clin Oncol 15(5):292–309
3. Halcrow PW, Dancer M, Panteah M et al (2016) Molecular changes associated with tumor initiation and progression of soft tissue sarcomas: targeting the genome and epigenome. Prog Mol Biol Transl Sci 144:323–380
4. Strauss DC, Hayes AJ, Thomas JM (2011) Retroperitoneal tumours: review of management. Ann R Coll Surg Engl 93(4):275–280
5. Porpiglia AS, Reddy SS, Farma JM (2016) Retroperitoneal sarcomas. Surg Clin North Am 96(5):993–1001
6. Clark MA, Fisher C, Judson I, Thomas JM (2005) Soft-tissue sarcomas in adults. N Engl J Med 353(7):701–711
7. Soini Y (2016) Epigenetic and genetic changes in soft tissue sarcomas: a review. APMIS 124(11):925–934
8. Sigston EAW, Williams BRG (2017) An emergence framework of carcinogenesis. Front Oncol 7:198
9. Gérard C, Goldbeter A (2016) Dynamics of the mammalian cell cycle in physiological and pathological conditions. Wiley Interdiscip Rev Syst Biol Med 8(2):140–156
10. Grizzi F, Chiriva-Internati M (2006) Cancer: looking for simplicity and finding complexity. Cancer Cell Int 6:4
11. Sell S, Nicolini A, Ferrari P, Biava PM (2016) Cancer: a problem of developmental biology; scientific evidence for reprogramming and differentiation therapy. Curr Drug Targets 17(10):1103–1110
12. Segal NH, Pavlidis P, Antonescu CR et al (2003) Classification and subtype prediction of adult soft tissue sarcoma by functional genomics. Am J Pathol 163(2):691–700
13. Strong LC, Williams WR, Tainsky MA (1992) The Li-Fraumeni syndrome: from clinical epidemiology to molecular genetics. Am J Epidemiol 135(2):190–199
14. Stratton MR, Moss S, Warren W et al (1990) Mutation of the p53 gene in human soft tissue sarcomas: association with abnormalities of the RB1 gene. Oncogene 5(9):1297–1301
15. Kruzelock RP, Hansen MF (1995) Molecular genetics and cytogenetics of sarcomas. Hematol Oncol Clin North Am 9(3):513–540
16. Skapek SX, Chui CH (2000) Cytogenetics and the biologic basis of sarcomas. Curr Opin Oncol 12(4):315–322
17. Karpeh MS, Brennan MF, Cance WG et al (1995) Altered patterns of retinoblastoma gene product expression in adult soft-tissue sarcomas. Br J Cancer 72(4):986–991
18. Xiao X, Garbutt CC, Hornicek F et al (2018) Advances in chromosomal translocations and fusion genes in sarcomas and potential therapeutic applications. Cancer Treat Rev 63:61–70
19. Jones KB (2018) What's in a name? Cell fate reprogramming in sarcomagenesis. Cancer Cell 33(1):5–7

20. Drummond CJ, Hanna JA, Garcia MR et al (2018) Hedgehog pathway drives fusion-negative rhabdomyosarcoma initiated from non-myogenic endothelial progenitors. Cancer Cell 33(1):108–124.e5
21. Oda Y, Yamamoto H, Kohashi K et al (2017) Soft tissue sarcomas: from a morphological to a molecular biological approach. Pathol Int 67(9):435–446
22. Hamacher R, Bauer S (2017) Preclinical models for translational sarcoma research. Curr Opin Oncol 29(4):275–285
23. Ramón y Cajal S, Castellvi J, Hümmer S et al (2018) Beyond molecular tumor heterogeneity: protein synthesis takes control. Oncogene 37(19):2490–2501
24. Chowell D, Napier J, Gupta R et al (2018) Modeling the subclonal evolution of cancer cell populations. Cancer Res 78(3):830–839
25. Greaves M, Maley CC (2012) Clonal evolution in cancer. Nature 481(7381):306–313
26. Osman S, Lehnert BE, Elojeimy S et al (2013) A comprehensive review of the retroperitoneal anatomy, neoplasms, and pattern of disease spread. Curr Probl Diagn Radiol 42(5):191–208
27. Loewenstein S, Lubezky N, Nizri E et al (2016) Adipose-induced retroperitoneal soft tissue sarcoma tumorigenesis: a potential crosstalk between sarcoma and fat cells. Mol Cancer Res 14(12):1254–1265
28. Grizzi F, Chiriva-Internati M (2005) The complexity of anatomical systems. Theor Biol Med Model 2:26
29. Ogino J, Asanuma H, Hatanaka Y et al (2013) Validity and reproducibility of Ki-67 assessment in gastrointestinal stromal tumors and leiomyosarcomas. Pathol Int 63(2):102–107
30. Ehnman M, Larsson O (2015) Microenvironmental targets in sarcoma. Front Oncol 5:248
31. Tomlinson J, Barsky SH, Nelson S et al (1999) Different patterns of angiogenesis in sarcomas and carcinomas. Clin Cancer Res 5(11):3516–3522
32. West CC, Brown NJ, Mangham DC et al (2005) Microvessel density does not predict outcome in high grade soft tissue sarcoma. Eur J Surg Oncol 31(10):1198–1205
33. D'Angelo SP, Shoushtari AN, Agaram NP et al (2015) Prevalence of tumor-infiltrating lymphocytes and PD-L1 expression in the soft tissue sarcoma microenvironment. Hum Pathol 46(3):357–365
34. Berghuis D, Santos SJ, Baelde HJ et al (2011) Pro-inflammatory chemokine-chemokine receptor interactions within the Ewing sarcoma microenvironment determine CD8(+) T-lymphocyte infiltration and affect tumour progression. J Pathol 223(3):347–357
35. Sorbye SW, Kilvaer T, Valkov A et al (2011) Prognostic impact of lymphocytes in soft tissue sarcomas. PLoS One 6(1):e14611
36. Tseng WW, Demicco EG, Lazar AJ et al (2012) Lymphocyte composition and distribution in inflammatory, well-differentiated retroperitoneal liposarcoma: clues to a potential adaptive immune response and therapeutic implications. Am J Surg Pathol 36(6):941–944
37. Blees A, Januliene D, Hofmann T et al (2017) Structure of the human MHC-I peptide-loading complex. Nature 551(7681):525–528
38. Berghuis D, de Hooge AS, Santos SJ et al (2009) Reduced human leukocyte antigen expression in advanced-stage Ewing sarcoma: implications for immune recognition. J Pathol 218(2):222–231
39. Garcia-Lora A, Martinez M, Algarra I et al (2003) MHC class I-deficient metastatic tumor variants immunoselected by T lymphocytes originate from the coordinated downregulation of APM components. Int J Cancer 106(4):521–527
40. Dunn GP, Bruce AT, Ikeda H et al (2002) Cancer immunoediting: from immunosurveillance to tumor escape. Nat Immunol 3(11):991–998
41. Leone P, Shin EC, Perosa F et al (2013) MHC class I antigen processing and presenting machinery: organization, function, and defects in tumor cells. J Natl Cancer Inst 105(16):1172–1187

42. Bukur J, Jasinski S, Seliger B (2012) The role of classical and non-classical HLA class I antigens in human tumors. Semin Cancer Biol 22(4):350–358

43. del Campo AB, Carretero J, Aptsiauri N, Garrido F (2012) Targeting HLA class I expression to increase tumor immunogenicity. Tissue Antigens 79(3):147–154

44. Seliger B, Ritz U, Ferrone S (2006) Molecular mechanisms of HLA class I antigen abnormalities following viral infection and transformation. Int J Cancer 118(1):129–138

45. Heemels MT, Ploegh H (1995) Generation, translocation, and presentation of MHC class I-restricted peptides. Annu Rev Biochem 64:463–491

46. Ortmann B, Copeman J, Lehner PJ et al (1997) A critical role for tapasin in the assembly and function of multimeric MHC class I-TAP complexes. Science 277(5330):1306–1309

47. Lehner PJ, Surman MJ, Cresswell P (1998) Soluble tapasin restores MHC class I expression and function in the tapasin-negative cell line .220. Immunity 8(2):221–231

48. Pamer E, Cresswell P (1998) Mechanisms of MHC class I–restricted antigen processing. Annu Rev Immunol 16:323–358

49. Peh CA, Burrows SR, Barnden M et al (1998) HLA-B27-restricted antigen presentation in the absence of tapasin reveals polymorphism in mechanisms of HLA class I peptide loading. Immunity 8(5):531–542

50. Barnden MJ, Purcell AW, Gorman JJ, McCluskey J (2000) Tapasin-mediated retention and optimization of peptide ligands during the assembly of class I molecules. J Immunol 165(1):322–330

51. Garbi N, Tan P, Diehl AD et al (2000) Impaired immune responses and altered peptide repertoire in tapasin-deficient mice. Nat Immunol 1(3):234–238

52. Grandea AG 3rd, Golovina TN, Hamilton SE et al (2000) Impaired assembly yet normal trafficking of MHC class I molecules in tapasin mutant mice. Immunity 13(2):213–222

53. Purcell AW, Gorman JJ, Garcia-Peydro M et al (2001) Quantitative and qualitative influences of tapasin on the class I peptide repertoire. J Immunol 166(2):1016–1027

54. Ogino T, Bandoh N, Hayashi T et al (2003) Association of tapasin and HLA class I antigen down-regulation in primary maxillary sinus squamous cell carcinoma lesions with reduced survival of patients. Clin Cancer Res 9(11):4043–4051

55. Anichini A, Mortarini R, Nonaka D et al (2006) Association of antigen-processing machinery and HLA antigen phenotype of melanoma cells with survival in American Joint Committee on Cancer stage III and IV melanoma patients. Cancer Res 66(12):6405–6411

56. Liu Y, Komohara Y, Domenick N et al (2012) Expression of antigen processing and presenting molecules in brain metastasis of breast cancer. Cancer Immunol Immunother 61(6):789–801

57. Seliger B (2008) Molecular mechanisms of MHC class I abnormalities and APM components in human tumors. Cancer Immunol Immunother 57(11):1719–1726

58. Ogino T, Shigyo H, Ishii H et al (2006) HLA class I antigen down-regulation in primary laryngeal squamous cell carcinoma lesions as a poor prognostic marker. Cancer Res 66(18):9281–9289

59. Campoli M, Chang CC, Ferrone S (2002) HLA class I antigen loss, tumor immune escape and immune selection. Vaccine 20(Suppl 4):A40–A45

60. Seliger B, Cabrera T, Garrido F, Ferrone S (2002) HLA class I antigen abnormalities and immune escape by malignant cells. Semin Cancer Biol 12(1):3–13

61. Chang CC, Campoli M, Ferrone S (2003) HLA class I defects in malignant lesions: what have we learned? Keio J Med 52(4):220–229

62. Atkins D, Ferrone S, Schmahl GE et al (2004) Down-regulation of HLA class I antigen processing molecules: an immune escape mechanism of renal cell carcinoma? J Urol 171(2 Pt 1):885–889

63. Campoli M, Chang CC, Oldford SA et al (2004) HLA antigen changes in malignant tumors of mammary epithelial origin: molecular mechanisms and clinical implications. Breast Dis 20:105–125

64. Facoetti A, Nano R, Zelini P et al (2005) Human leukocyte antigen and antigen processing machinery component defects in astrocytic tumors. Clin Cancer Res 11(23):8304–8311
65. Ferris RL, Hunt JL, Ferrone S (2005) Human leukocyte antigen (HLA) class I defects in head and neck cancer: molecular mechanisms and clinical significance. Immunol Res 33(2):113–133
66. Kloor M, Becker C, Benner A et al (2005) Immunoselective pressure and human leukocyte antigen class I antigen machinery defects in microsatellite unstable colorectal cancers. Cancer Res 65(14):6418–6424
67. Meissner M, Reichert TE, Kunkel M et al (2005) Defects in the human leukocyte antigen class I antigen processing machinery in head and neck squamous cell carcinoma: association with clinical outcome. Clin Cancer Res 11(7):2552–2560
68. Raffaghello L, Prigione I, Bocca P et al (2005) Multiple defects of the antigen-processing machinery components in human neuroblastoma: immunotherapeutic implications. Oncogene 24(29):4634–4644
69. Vitale M, Pelusi G, Taroni B et al (2005) HLA class I antigen down-regulation in primary ovary carcinoma lesions: association with disease stage. Clin Cancer Res 11(1):67–72
70. Bangia N, Ferrone S (2006) Antigen presentation machinery (APM) modulation and soluble HLA molecules in the tumor microenvironment: do they provide tumor cells with escape mechanisms from recognition by cytotoxic T lymphocytes? Immunol Invest 35(3–4):485–503
71. Chang CC, Ogino T, Mullins DW et al (2006) Defective human leukocyte antigen class I-associated antigen presentation caused by a novel beta2-microglobulin loss-of-function in melanoma cells. J Biol Chem 281(27):18763–18773
72. Ferris RL, Whiteside TL, Ferrone S (2006) Immune escape associated with functional defects in antigen-processing machinery in head and neck cancer. Clin Cancer Res 12(13):3890–3895
73. López-Albaitero A, Nayak JV, Ogino T et al (2006) Role of antigen-processing machinery in the in vitro resistance of squamous cell carcinoma of the head and neck cells to recognition by CTL. J Immunol 176(6):3402–3409
74. Chang CC, Ferrone S (2007) Immune selective pressure and HLA class I antigen defects in malignant lesions. Cancer Immunol Immunother 56(2):227–236
75. Seliger B, Stoehr R, Handke D et al (2010) Association of HLA class I antigen abnormalities with disease progression and early recurrence in prostate cancer. Cancer Immunol Immunother 59(4):529–540
76. Campoli M, Ferrone S (2008) HLA antigen changes in malignant cells: epigenetic mechanisms and biologic significance. Oncogene 27(45):5869–5885
77. del Campo AB, Kyte JA, Carretero J et al (2014) Immune escape of cancer cells with beta2-microglobulin loss over the course of metastatic melanoma. Int J Cancer 134(1):102–113
78. Fairweather M, Gonzalez RJ, Strauss D, Raut CP (2018) Current principles of surgery for retroperitoneal sarcomas. J Surg Oncol 117(1):33–41
79. Segal NH, Blachere NE, Guevara-Patiño JA et al (2005) Identification of cancer-testis genes expressed by melanoma and soft tissue sarcoma using bioinformatics. Cancer Immun 5(1):2
80. Roszik J, Wang WL, Livingston JA et al (2017) Overexpressed PRAME is a potential immunotherapy target in sarcoma subtypes. Clin Sarcoma Res 7:11
81. Pollack SM, Ingham M, Spraker MB, Schwartz GK (2018) Emerging targeted and immune-based therapies in sarcoma. J Clin Oncol 36(2):125–135
82. Salmaninejad A, Zamani MR, Pourvahedi M et al (2016) Cancer/testis antigens: expression, regulation, tumor invasion, and use in immunotherapy of cancers. Immunol Invest 45(7):619–640
83. Chiriva-Internati M, Grizzi F, Bright RK, Martin Kast W (2004) Cancer immunotherapy: avoiding the road to perdition. J Transl Med 2(1):26

84. Iura K, Maekawa A, Kohashi K et al (2017) Cancer-testis antigen expression in synovial sarcoma: NY-ESO-1, PRAME, MAGEA4, and MAGEA1. Hum Pathol 61:130–139
85. Iura K, Kohashi K, Hotokebuchi Y et al (2015) Cancer-testis antigens PRAME and NY-ESO-1 correlate with tumour grade and poor prognosis in myxoid liposarcoma. J Pathol Clin Res 1(3):144–159
86. Iura K, Kohashi K, Ishii T et al (2017) MAGEA4 expression in bone and soft tissue tumors: its utility as a target for immunotherapy and diagnostic marker combined with NY-ESO-1. Virchows Arch 471(3):383–392
87. Groisberg R, Hong DS, Behrang A et al (2017) Characteristics and outcomes of patients with advanced sarcoma enrolled in early phase immunotherapy trials. J Immunother Cancer 5(1):100
88. Zheng B, Ren T, Huang Y, Guo W (2018) Apatinib inhibits migration and invasion as well as PD-L1 expression in osteosarcoma by targeting STAT3. Biochem Biophys Res Commun 495(2):1695–1701
89. Machado I, López-Guerrero JA, Scotlandi K et al (2018) Immunohistochemical analysis and prognostic significance of PD-L1, PD-1, and CD8+ tumor-infiltrating lymphocytes in Ewing's sarcoma family of tumors (ESFT). Virchows Arch 472(5):815–824
90. Boxberg M, Steiger K, Lenze U et al (2018) PD-L1 and PD-1 and characterization of tumor-infiltrating lymphocytes in high grade sarcomas of soft tissue – prognostic implications and rationale for immunotherapy. Oncoimmunology 7(3):e1389366
91. Zhu Z, Jin Z, Zhang M et al (2017) Prognostic value of programmed death-ligand 1 in sarcoma: a meta-analysis. Oncotarget 8(35):59570–59580

Imaging of Retroperitoneal Sarcomas

4

Luca Balzarini, Nicolò Gennaro, and Carlo Morosi

4.1 Diseases

Retroperitoneal soft tissue sarcomas (RPS) are rare and account for approximately 12–15% of all soft tissue sarcomas, with a mean incidence of 2.7 per million. The peak incidence occurs during the fifth decade of life [1–3] and these tumors represent a third of retroperitoneal tumors.

In the adult, more frequent conditions include primary lymphoproliferative disease, parenchymatous epithelial tumors and metastases (germ cell tumors, carcinomas and melanomas), whereas Wilms' tumor, neuroblastoma and germ cell tumor are the most frequent conditions affecting the young patient. The understanding of the normal anatomy and the comprehensive assessment of the retroperitoneal space, along with a good familiarity with retroperitoneal diseases and patterns of spread, are critical to the radiologist when suspecting a RPS [4]. The retroperitoneal space is one of the most difficult regions to assess due to the multiplicity of fascial layers, spaces and interfascial planes contained within it. The anatomy of the retroperitoneum, owing to the loose connective tissue also explains why these tumors tend to grow undisturbed until gastrointestinal, urinary or neurovascular involvement occurs [5].

4.2 Imaging in the Management of Retroperitoneal Sarcoma

4.2.1 Role of Imaging

Diagnostic imaging represents the cornerstone of RPS proper management, which can be differentiated in the following steps: identification, location, differential

L. Balzarini (✉)
Department of Radiology, Humanitas Clinical and Research Center
Rozzano, Milan, Italy
e-mail: luca.balzarini@humanitas.it

V. Quagliuolo, A. Gronchi (Eds), *Current Treatment of Retroperitoneal Sarcomas*, 33
Updates in Surgery
DOI: 10.1007/978-88-470-3980-3_4, © Springer-Verlag Italia 2019

diagnosis, staging, biopsy guidance, monitoring of treatment response and eventually restaging, follow-up.

Clear and standardized communication between radiologists and dedicated multidisciplinary teams allows for a comprehensive clinical, histopathological, and radiological assessment, a pivotal effort prior to surgical resection, whose completeness is still the most important factor in long-term survival [6]. Due to their rarity and the challenges that surgery and imaging have to face when assessing retroperitoneal masses, RPS must be invariably referred to high-volume centers where an improved prognosis has been demonstrated [7].

4.2.2   Radiographs

Conventional radiography has a limited role in the staging and follow-up of RPS. Conventional radiography identifies calcifications inside the tumor and any adjacent bone involvement.

4.2.3   Ultrasound

Ultrasonography (US) is a well-known, inexpensive and non-harming imaging method used to detect retroperitoneal masses. Modern probes with high spatial resolution provide a good depiction of retroperitoneal masses and can also be used as image guidance for biopsy. Moreover, US does not suffer from metallic implants that reduce the imaging quality in computed tomography and magnetic resonance imaging.

The limits of US are the low inter- and intra-observer agreement, low repeatability of the examination, patient habitus and the operator's technique-related skills. For these reasons, US is infrequently employed in the staging and follow-up of RPS.

4.2.4   Computed Tomography and Magnetic Resonance Imaging

Computed tomography (CT) and magnetic resonance imaging (MRI) nowadays are the modalities of choice to assess retroperitoneal masses. They play an important role in:
1. Identifying and characterizing the masses in terms of location, size and extension in the retroperitoneal space;
2. Drawing a spectrum of differential diagnosis (solid/cystic, neoplastic/non-neoplastic);
3. Guiding the percutaneous biopsy;
4. Planning the surgery to help achieve complete surgical resection through

the evaluation of local soft tissue infiltration and relationships with critical neurovascular structures;

5. Identifying postoperative complications;
6. Assessing response to neoadjuvant treatment;
7. Follow-up and restaging.

The first challenge for imaging is defining the location of the tumor. Since RPS account for only 30% of retroperitoneal masses, more common lesions have to be ruled out. In this regard, the displacement of normal anatomical structures is helpful. Anterior dislocation of kidneys, adrenal glands, pancreas, ascending and descending colon and middle portion of the duodenum or major vessels suggests a tumor arising from the retroperitoneal cavity.

A wide differential diagnosis based on anatomical relationship, CT attenuation and MRI signal intensity has then to be started. Unfortunately, imaging is not capable of distinguishing between more than 50 varieties of histological RPS subtypes [8], even if the majority of RPS can be summarized into liposarcomas (70%) and leiomyosarcomas (15%), which do present some typical features on imaging. Although in a few fat-containing RPS (well-differentiated and dedifferentiated liposarcomas) the radiologist may be able to make a confident diagnosis, biopsy is usually mandatory to confirm and characterize the radiological findings.

The anatomical relationships of RPS are well-depicted by cross-sectional imaging like contrast-enhanced CT and MRI. CT, which is widely available, provides a superior spatial resolution and an accurate detection of calcifications. Contrast-enhanced CT is the appropriate choice for assessing vascular and visceral involvement, including secondary lesions, usually in the liver and the lung. MRI, because of its higher soft tissue contrast resolution, is of great utility when the pelvis is involved, during follow-up and every time CT is insufficient to provide the surgeon with critical information about local tumor extent. Moreover, if bone, muscles or foramina are involved, MRI should be the method of choice.

MRI gives structural information through a precise assessment of the fat component inside the mass, of the internal necrotic areas and of the surrounding edema. It can be useful in delineating tissue planes and determining the organ of origin and the spread of the disease, allowing for a more accurate diagnosis and staging.

MRI plays also a critical role during follow-up when differentiation has to be made between postsurgical soft tissues changes and local recurrence. Vanel et al. described that the presence of low signal intensity on T2-weighted MRI had 96% sensitivity for excluding the presence of recurrence [9]. However, after surgical treatment a few different non-neoplastic tissues can be present, including fatty atrophy, seroma or inflammatory change. These findings can show a high signal intensity in fluid-sensitive sequences at conventional MRI, mimicking signs of recurrence. Dynamic gadolinium-enhanced MR imaging can help to differentiate recurrent tumor from an inflammatory pseudotumor. Recurrence tends to enhance during the early arterial phase, whereas pseudotumors tend to enhance in late venous phase (Fig. 4.4). Diffusion-weighted imaging (DWI) is also useful to distinguish tumor and recurrence because of the high restriction of water diffusion due to high cellularity of the malignant mass, resulting in high signal intensity. Finally, in patients with allergy to iodinated contrast agent, MRI remains the only solution to substitute CT.

Since complete resection of the mass (R0) is the mainstay of RPS treatment, detailed description of the radiological findings are required to plan a radical treatment. The radiological report must include the precise location, the anatomic relationships with neurovascular structures and viscera, the tumor extent and the multifocality of the disease, whenever present (12%) [2].

Frequent causes of non-resectability are peritoneal implants, distant metastases or involvement of vascular structures, or multifocality. The extent of any involvement of the inferior vena cava or major trunk vessels, as well as any intraluminal component has to be accurately reported. Sometimes resectability looks feasible due to the presence of a pseudocapsule, but this can simply be represented by the compressed tissue of surrounding organs.

In the case of large vessel involvement, CT and MRI are useful to quantify the extent of the vascular encasement (tumor involvement >180°) or effacement (<180°, without change of caliber) and to identify intraluminal thrombus. In fact, compressed venous vessels increase the risk for venous thromboembolism and the pulmonary vascularization should always be checked to rule out pulmonary embolism [10].

4.2.5   Hybrid Imaging

Fluorine-18 deoxyglucose positron emission tomography (PET)/CT (FDG PET/CT) has no clear role for the diagnosis of RPS. Although it can detect primary and recurrent soft tissue lesions, discrimination between low-grade tumors and benign lesions is rather poor [11]. FDG PET may play a role in defining the spread of neoplasm, to exclude pulmonary metastasis or multifocal intra-abdominal disease and to assess early treatment response. FDG PET/CT may be used to help guide biopsy toward the most FDG-avid component of the tumor.

PET/MRI represents the next challenge for hybrid imaging, consisting in a logistical, time-saving advantage and non-harming imaging system for the patient. However, hybrid systems still need to be evaluated in prospective studies.

4.3 Radiological Findings in Retroperitoneal Sarcomas

4.3.1 Liposarcoma

Adipocytic tumors represent the widest part of the spectrum of RPS in patients over 55 years old. The presence of fat is easily recognized owing to its attenuation on CT or its high signal on T1- and T2-weighted MRI, with a characteristic loss of signal intensity in fat-suppressed sequences. Liposarcoma presents with a large-sized, well-rounded mass, with homogeneous fatty content in the case of well-differentiated liposarcomas (WDLPS). Nevertheless, up to 50% do not have detectable fat inside, and US, CT and MRI have consequently a non-specific appearance [12].

Adipocytic tumors are classified only after pathological analysis, based on the most aggressive cellular components within the specimen. Liposarcoma can be locally aggressive (well-differentiated) with the following subtypes: lipoma–like, sclerosing, round cell, inflammatory and spindle–cell like. Malignant adipocytic tumors are classified as myxoid, pleomorphic, dedifferentiated or not otherwise specified (NOS) liposarcomas (Fig. 4.1). Different histological subtypes may frequently coexist in the same lesion (Fig. 4.1a). It is vital to recognize that the absence of macroscopic fat in the retroperitoneal mass does not exclude a WDLPS (like the sclerosing subtype). The radiological findings are very similar to those of subcutaneous fat or those of simple lipoma. Smooth margins with lobular contours, thick septa (<3 mm), and a nodular component with low contrast enhancement are usually present (Fig. 4.1). The possible extension of tumors outside the abdominal cavity through the diaphragmatic hiatus, inguinal canal, sciatic notch or obturator foramen should be described for surgical planning. Although rare in the retroperitoneum, benign fat-containing masses such as extragonadal dermoids, hibernomas, extramedullary hematopoiesis and lipomas can mimic WDLPS.

Dedifferentiated liposarcomas (DDLPS) are high grade tumors. Characteristic findings include a non-lipomatous mass surrounded by a fatty mass, even though evidence of fat is lacking in up to 20% of cases. Calcifications can be present and usually indicate dedifferentiation and therefore poor prognosis. Calcifications are typically found also in the sclerosing or inflammatory variant of WDLPS (Fig. 4.1c) [13, 14]. Characteristic nodular or irregularly linear septa (>2 mm wide) within the lesion enhance markedly after intravenous contrast medium administration. Unfortunately, a rigorous differential diagnosis between DDLPS and WDLPS cannot be always performed on the basis of imaging alone, even after contrast administration. Myxoid and pleomorphic liposarcomas are rarely found in the retroperitoneum.

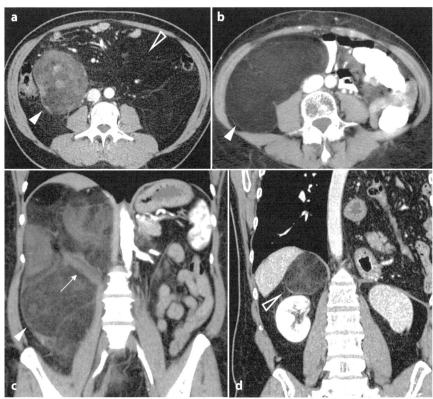

Fig. 4.1 Fatty lesions of the retroperitoneum. **a** Concomitant presence of well-differentiated (*black arrowhead*) and dedifferentiated (*white arrowhead*) liposarcomas in the same patient. **b** Lipoma-like liposarcoma arising within the right perirenal space (*white arrowhead*). **c** Sclerosing-type well-differentiated liposarcoma arising within the right posterior pararenal space (*white arrowhead*), with fibrotic septa within the lesion (*arrow*). **d** Myelolipoma of the adrenal gland in the right perirenal space (*black arrowhead*)

4.3.2   Leiomyosarcoma

Leiomyosarcoma accounts for 15% of RPS, thus representing the most common RPS in the young and the second most common RPS among adults. It originates from the smooth muscle in the wall of retroperitoneal veins or from the Wolffian remnants. Most commonly, leiomyosarcoma arises from the inferior vena cava below the level of the hepatic veins, but also renal or gonadal veins can be involved (Fig. 4.2). Leiomyosarcomas are more common in women in the 5th and 6th decade and can be either extravascular-extraluminal (62%), extravascular-intraluminal (33%) or rarely intravascular-intraluminal. A large, lobulated, heterogeneously enhancing, necrotic retroperitoneal mass contiguous with a vessel, with same appearance of that of the muscle, is highly suspicious of a leiomyosarcoma.

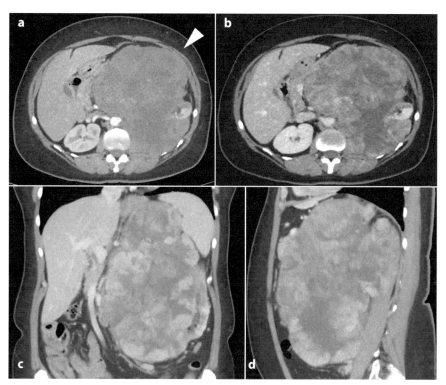

Fig. 4.2 Leiomyosarcoma. Contrast-enhanced computed tomography shows a high-grade leiomyosarcoma (*arrowhead*) originating from the left renal hilum involving the left kidney, adrenal gland, pancreas and spleen, with dislocation of vascular and visceral structures. **a** Arterial phase, axial; **b** venous phase, axial; **c** venous phase, coronal; **d** venous phase, sagittal

The presence of intraluminal components helps to differentiate leiomyosarcoma from other retroperitoneal masses and an exophytic component mimicking an extrinsic compression on the vessel can be found [15]. Leiomyosarcoma is highly metastasizing, with metastases already present at time of the initial diagnosis in 40% of cases [16, 17]. CT findings are those of a large mass with well-defined margins, isoattenuating to muscle; at MRI the signal intensity is heterogeneously low-to-intermediate on T1-weighted scans and intermediate-to-high on T2-weighted scans with internal areas of necrosis or cystic degeneration. After contrast enhancement, arterial phase imaging well depicts the feeding vessels and shows a typical peripheral pattern of enhancement.

4.3.3. Solitary Fibrous Tumors

Solitary fibrous tumors represent the third commonest variant of RPS, which have been shown to arise from any site of the body, most frequent in the thorax.

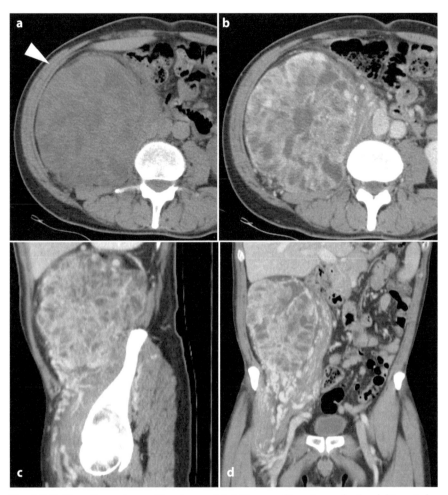

Fig. 4.3 Solitary fibrous tumor. Pseudocapsulated fibrous solitary tumor in the right posterior pararenal space (*arrowheads*) without visceral involvement. Contrast-enhanced computed tomography acquisitions show extensive contrast enhancement in every phase with enlarged venous vessels arising from the mass. **a** Non-contrast-enhanced image, axial; **b** venous phase, axial; **c** venous phase, sagittal; **d** venous phase, coronal

Most hemangiopericytomas are now classified as solitary fibrous tumors in the updated WHO classification of soft tissue tumors, which re-classified many diseases according to breakthroughs in molecular genetics.

These tumors appear as well–defined, hypervascular masses, with heterogeneous findings in terms of attenuation (CT) and MRI signal. In the delayed phase, an intense contrast enhancement due to the fibrous stroma is described (Fig. 4.3). Rare calcifications, areas of necrosis, hemorrhage or cystic changes are usually seen.

4.3.4 Malignant Peripheral Nerve Sheath Tumor

Malignant peripheral nerve sheath tumors (MPNSTs) are soft tissue tumors originating from Schwann cells and characterized by local invasion and a potential for metastasizing. They can arise de novo or from a preexisting neurofibroma, as in the setting of neurofibromatosis type 1 (50% of cases) [18]. Usually they arise in the sciatic nerve, brachial or sacral plexus, but they can also take origin from the retroperitoneum or in the extremities. The lesions appear hypodense at non-enhanced CT, with an early and peripheral pattern of enhancement after iodide contrast administration. The MRI signal is non-specific and non-homogeneous, with a propensity to show iso-hypointensity on T1-weighted scans and hyperintensity on T2-weighted scans. Cystic degeneration and lack of capsulation is usually described. The differential diagnosis with benign peripheral nerve sheath tumors (BPNSTs) can be challenging, since there is no single radiological feature capable of discriminating between a benign plexiform variant and a malignant nerve sheath tumor. When rhabdomyoblastic differentiation is noted, MPNSTs are referred to as malignant tritons. Like undifferentiated sarcomas, some MPNSTs (10%) are secondary to radiation therapy [19].

4.3.5 Undifferentiated Sarcomas

A consistent part of undifferentiated sarcomas arises in the context of retro-peritoneal muscles (i.e., iliopsoas). They may be secondary to local radiation therapy [16].

Imaging characteristics are non-specific and the differential diagnosis is challenging [20]. In CT imaging, they present as a well-circumscribed mass, iso-hypoattenuated to muscle, with heterogeneous content due to foci of necrosis, hemorrhage, and myxoid area. A nodular or peripheral pattern of the enhancement can be visualized after contrast medium administration and calcifications are frequent (up to 20%). Direct invasion into adjacent organs may also be present. MRI is non-specific, with heterogeneous signal intensity on all pulse sequences, which usually consists of hypo-iso-intensity signal on T1-weighted scans and iso-hyperintense signal in T2-weighted scans. The margins may appear well-defined with a classic fibrotic pseudocapsule with low signal intensity in both on T1- and T2-weighted scans, calcifications, hemorrhage and necrosis. The solid component within the lesion shows a typical peripheral nodular pattern of enhancement after contrast administration.

4.3.6 Desmoid Tumor

Also known as deep fibromatosis (singular or multiple), desmoid tumor is a locally aggressive lesion consisting of fibroblastic proliferation without inflammation that destroys soft tissue planes.

Typical findings of this tumor are an infiltrative mass with heterogeneous attenuation at CT and variable MRI signal (usually starting with a high signal intensity on T2-weighted scans) which fades later when cellularity decreases in favor of collagen deposition. Nevertheless, differentiating this tumor from other sarcomas is challenging, especially in the differential diagnosis with undifferentiated sarcomas.

4.3.7 Perivascular Epithelioid Cell Tumor

Perivascular epithelioid cell tumors (PEComas) are mesenchymal tumors of varying malignant potential. They are often indistinguishable from retroperitoneal masses like angiomyolipoma, lymphangioleiomyomatosis or pigmented melanotic tumors.

4.3.8 Synovial Sarcoma

Synovial sarcoma is a malignant tumor which can be found rarely in the retroperitoneum. Imaging findings are non-specific, showing a hypodense mass on CT and heterogeneous signal intensity on MRI with a peripheral contrast enhancement and central necrosis.

4.3.9 Myelolipoma

Myelolipoma is a benign tumor that consists of mature adipocytes and hematopoietic components. It rarely arises outside the adrenal glands (15%), usually in the presacral space and in the retroperitoneum. A typical radiological finding is a predominant fat-containing mass similar to liposarcoma, with low contrast enhancement in both early and delayed phase (Fig. 4.1d).

4.4 Core-Needle Biopsy of Retroperitoneal Sarcomas: How and When

Due to the impossibility of establishing a definitive diagnosis on an imaging basis only, pathological assessment remains the mainstay of diagnosis. An early definitive diagnosis allows for a clear distinction between RPS and retroperitoneal malignant (lymphomas, metastases and primary carcinomas) and benign lesions. Image-guided biopsy should be performed after consultation with a multidisciplinary team dedicated to soft tissue tumors for appropriate planning. Only some WDLPS and DDLPS with typical radiological findings can be confidentially diagnosed on cross-sectional imaging without sample analysis. When neoadjuvant therapy is not indicated, the lesion can be resected en bloc with no need for preoperative biopsy.

Three kinds of specimens can be obtained: cytological (fine-needle aspiration cytology), histological (core needle biopsy) and gross pathological specimen (surgical incisional biopsy). Fine-needle aspiration cytology is not recommended since it rarely yields diagnostic information. Open or laparoscopic biopsy is expensive, exposes the peritoneal cavity to contamination and unnecessarily alters the anatomy before the surgical excisional procedure. Core needle biopsy, on the contrary, is a safe and feasible procedure that does not negatively influence the oncological outcome of patients [21].

Image-guidance is always recommended, even if the tumor is large and palpable, to prevent inadvertent damage to adjacent structures and avoid cystic or necrotic area inside the tumor. Among the methods available to provide a proper specimen for analysis, a percutaneous, CT-guided core needle biopsy with coaxial biopsy needles (14–16 G) is the modality of choice. Compared to fine needle aspiration cytology, core needle biopsy provides enough tissue not just for morphological analysis but also for immunohistochemistry, genetic, and molecular analysis.

The optimal route is the retroperitoneal approach, preserving the posterior parietal peritoneum, which shows a minimal risk of seeding (0.37%) [21]. At least three biopsy specimens of what appears the most aggressive-appearing portion of the lesion should be available to establish the type and grade through histologic and molecular subtyping. When it is not possible to perform percutaneous biopsy, in rare circumstances histological samples can be obtained under endoscopic ultrasound guidance.

4.5 Differential Diagnosis

Imaging cannot be used to predict the cell types of most common retroperitoneal sarcomas except typical cases of liposarcomas. The gold standard still remains histopathological analysis that has recently updated the overall classifications of sarcomas due to the recent advances of immunochemistry [22]. More exact diagnoses depend on recent advances in immunohistochemistry assays, which allow defining the subtypes of tumors based on cell surface markers better than histology alone.

A major task for the radiologist is to discriminate between malignant and benign disease, which account only for the 10–20% of primary retroperitoneal tumors. In most cases, based on clinical history and radiological findings it is possible to distinguish between benign mass, reactive, inflammatory and infectious conditions from malignant tumors.

Retroperitoneal tumors are subdivided into mesodermal, neurogenic and extragonadal germ tumors. The differential diagnosis includes tumor arising from retroperitoneal viscera (pancreas, duodenum, adrenal glands and kidneys), lymphoma or metastatic lesion (testicles). The prevalence of fat content and soft tissues inside the mass generally indicates a low-grade tumor whereas dedifferentiated lesions are more likely to be infiltrative, heterogeneous and hypervascularized.

On the contrary, heterogeneous signal intensity at MRI and hemorrhage have been shown to be poor prognostic features. A recent study by Lahat et al. examined the possibility for CT to perform the histologic classification of liposarcomas based on characteristics such as their percentage of fat, definition of limits, focal nodular/water density, ground glass opacities and hypervascularity, showing that typical cases of WDLPS should not be biopsied [14]. Imaging can rely on laboratory and clinical data to orient the differential diagnosis, searching for a previous history of malignancy or positive serum markers for other primary tumors (ectopic testicular tumors have to be ruled out with ultrasound) and excludes retroperitoneal fibrosis especially after bilateral ureteral involvement.

Retroperitoneal fibrosis (RPF) is a rare fibrotic process that typically originates at the level of lumbosacral vertebrae and tends to extend superiorly in a periaortic and perivascular distribution toward the renal hila. Typically, the middle third of ureters is encased, giving origin to a bilateral and symmetrical postrenal urinary obstruction. At CT imaging, RPF presents as a homogeneous mass with attenuation equivalent to soft tissue, whereas at MRI the signal is low-to-intermediate on both T1- and T2-weighted scans and varies depending on disease activity, which ranges from a chronic active inflammation phase (high signal intensity on T2-weighted MRI) to fibrous scarring (low signal intensity on T2-weighted MRI). The malignant subtype of RPF is unusual and generally presents as a more heterogeneous lesion, with moderate enhancement, poorly defined margins and a tendency to invasive spread with vertebral involvement.

RPS generally never spread to lymph nodes except rare cases of clear cell sarcoma, epithelioid sarcoma and rhabdomyosarcoma.

4.6   Follow-up

Despite complete resection, recurrent disease is the leading cause of death in RPS (Fig. 4.4). After surgical treatment, surveillance with contrast-enhanced CT

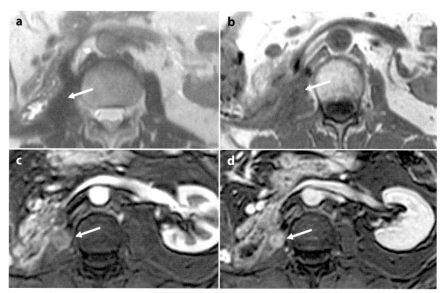

Fig. 4.4 Liposarcoma. Early recurrence of liposarcoma (*arrow*) in the right pararenal space after surgical resection. The recurrent nodule is well depicted in T1-weighted scans after contrast administration (early enhancement in the arterial phase). The nodule was not visible in unenhanced sequences. **a** T1-weighted MRI; **b** T2-weighted MRI; **c** arterial phase, contrast-enhanced T1-weighted MRI; **d** venous phase, contrast-enhanced T1-weighted MRI

of the chest, abdomen and pelvis is indicated to detect recurrence years before the clinical appearance of symptoms. Particularly important is the first check after treatment, which must exclude the presence of persistent foci of disease. It also represents the initial postoperative baseline imaging examination to be compared with further evaluations.

A strict follow-up needs therefore to be scheduled to promptly intercept local recurrences. Local recurrence is also positively associated with a high risk of distant metastasis (peritoneum, lung, abdominal viscera).

Current guidelines from ESMO/European Sarcoma Network Working Group published in 2014 [23] recommend for intermediate-high grade disease a contrast-enhanced CT scan of the chest, abdomen, and pelvis every 3–4 months for the first 2–3 years, then every 6 months until the fifth year, then annually. For low-grade disease, a CT has to be acquired every 4–6 months, with chest X-ray or CT scan at longer intervals in the first 3–5 years, then annually.

Annual monitoring up to 10 years is considered sufficient to detect any local recurrence or metastatic disease but, since the risk of recurrence never ends, a personalized follow-up should be scheduled for each patient. The huge amount of ionizing radiation required by this kind of follow-up protocol makes MRI an interesting solution for younger patients and to re-stage the abdomen and pelvis.

Evaluation of the surgical bed is challenging due to the presence of scarring and fibrosis. CT and MRI are considered the gold standard methods to monitor and restage RPS. The inherent soft tissue contrast of MRI is ideally well-suited for the assessment of soft tissue masses, and high signal intensity on T2-weighted scans and STIR sequences is typical of malignant masses [24]. However, seroma formation, fatty atrophy and postirradiation inflammatory change can mimic a high T2-signal intensity.

Ultrasound is an underutilized imaging method to assess recurrent sarcomas. They appear as low echogenic nodules with a round, oval or lobulated morphology. Its diagnostic performance has been compared to MRI in the detection of local recurrence of soft tissue sarcoma and both techniques were found to be equally useful [25].

Recurrent tumors tend to enhance at an earlier stage, usually within a few seconds (Fig. 4.4) [26]. Thus, dynamic gadolinium-enhanced MRI can help in the differentiation of recurrent tumor from an inflammatory pseudotumor (Fig. 4.4) [27]. Rapid initial and decrease enhancement curve and non-peripheral enhancement have also been described as markers of malignancy.

In recent studies, PET has been shown to be more sensitive than CT and MR imaging in the detection of recurrent and metastatic disease [28, 29].

4.7   Conclusions

The radiologist plays a vital role in establishing the diagnosis, defining extension and anatomical relationship of the mass, performing image-guided biopsy, staging the tumor and assessing the feasibility of curative surgery. CT is the most useful and widely available imaging modality in staging and restaging of RPS, whereas MRI is a problem-solving imaging method in terms of disease detection, characterization and anatomical definition.

Because of the large spectrum of lesions which can occur in the retroperitoneum, biopsy remains the standard diagnostic procedure. A correct histopathological diagnosis is critical in planning the most appropriate treatment approach, which needs to be performed in a specialized soft tissue sarcoma center.

References

1. Gronchi A, Strauss DC, Miceli R et al (2016) Variability in patterns of recurrence after resection of primary retroperitoneal sarcoma (RPS): a report on 1007 patients from the Multi-institutional Collaborative RPS Working Group. Ann Surg 263(5):1002–1009
2. Mullinax JE, Zager JS, Gonzalez RJ (2011) Current diagnosis and management of retroperitoneal sarcoma. Cancer Control 18(3):177–187

3. Bonvalot S, Rivoire M, Castaing M et al (2009) Primary retroperitoneal sarcomas: a multivariate analysis of surgical factors associated with local control. J Clin Oncol 27(1):31–37
4. Osman S, Lehnert BE, Elojeimy S et al (2013) A comprehensive review of the retroperitoneal anatomy, neoplasms, and pattern of disease spread. Curr Probl Diagn Radiol 42(5):191–208
5. Van Roggen JF, Hogendoorn PC (2000) Soft tissue tumours of the retroperitoneum. Sarcoma 4(1–2):17–26
6. Messiou C, Moskovic E, Vanel D et al (2017) Primary retroperitoneal soft tissue sarcoma: imaging appearances, pitfalls and diagnostic algorithm. Eur J Surg Oncol 43(7):1191–1198
7. Gutierrez JC, Perez EA, Moffat FL et al (2007) Should soft tissue sarcomas be treated at high-volume centers? An analysis of 4205 patients. Ann Surg 245(6):952–958
8. Morosi C, Stacchiotti S, Marchianò A et al (2014) Correlation between radiological assessment and histopathological diagnosis in retroperitoneal tumors: analysis of 291 consecutive patients at a tertiary reference sarcoma center. Eur J Surg Oncol 40(12):1662–1670
9. Vanel D, Lacombe MJ, Couanet D et al (1987) Musculoskeletal tumors: follow-up with MR imaging after treatment with surgery and radiation therapy. Radiology 164(1):243–245
10. Miah AB, Hannay J, Benson C et al (2014) Optimal management of primary retroperitoneal sarcoma: an update. Expert Rev Anticancer Ther 14(5):565–579
11. Ioannidis JPA, Lau J (2003) 18F-FDG PET for the diagnosis and grading of soft-tissue sarcoma: a meta-analysis. J Nucl Med 44(5):717–724
12. Hong SH, Kim KA, Woo OH et al (2010) Dedifferentiated liposarcoma of retroperitoneum: spectrum of imaging findings in 15 patients. Clin Imaging 34(3):203–210
13. Craig WD, Fanburg-Smith JC, Henry LR et al (2009) Fat-containing lesions of the retroperitoneum: radiologic-pathologic correlation. Radiographics 29(1):261–290
14. Lahat G, Madewell JE, Anaya DA et al (2009) Computed tomography scan-driven selection of treatment for retroperitoneal liposarcoma histologic subtypes. Cancer 115(5): 1081–1090
15. Ganeshalingam S, Rajeswaran G, Jones RL et al (2011) Leiomyosarcomas of the inferior vena cava: diagnostic features on cross-sectional imaging. Clin Radiol 66(1):50–56
16. Rajiah P, Sinha R, Cuevas C et al (2011) Imaging of uncommon retroperitoneal masses. Radiographics 31(4):949–976
17. O'Sullivan PJ, Harris AC, Munk PL (2008) Radiological imaging features of non-uterine leiomyosarcoma. Br J Radiol 81(961):73–81
18. Meis-Kindblom JM (1995) Color atlas of soft tissue tumors, 1st edn. Mosby-Wolfe, St Louis
19. Ducatman BS, Scheithauer BW, Piepgras DG et al (1986) Malignant peripheral nerve sheath tumors. A clinicopathologic study of 120 cases. Cancer 57(10):2006–2021
20. Lu J-H, Yang T, Yang G-S et al (2008) Retroperitoneal malignant fibrous histiocytoma mimicking hepatocellular carcinoma. Eur J Radiol Extra 65(3):91–96
21. Van Houdt WJ, Schrijver AM, Cohen-Hallaleh RB et al (2017) Needle tract seeding following core biopsies in retroperitoneal sarcoma. Eur J Surg Oncol 43(9):1740–1745
22. Baheti AD, O'Malley RB, Kim S et al (2016) Soft-tissue sarcomas: an update for radiologists based on the revised 2013 World Health Organization classification. AJR Am J Roentgenol 206(5):924–932
23. Casali PG, Abecassis N, Bauer S et al (2018) Soft tissue and visceral sarcomas: ESMO-EURACAN Clinical Practice Guidelines for diagnosis, treatment and follow-up. Ann Oncol [Epub ahead of print] doi:10.1093/annonc/mdy096
24. James SL, Davies AM (2008) Post-operative imaging of soft tissue sarcomas. Cancer Imaging 8(1):8–18
25. Choi H, Varma DG, Fornage BD et al (1991) Soft-tissue sarcoma: MR imaging vs sonography for detection of local recurrence after surgery. AJR Am J Roentgenol 157(2):353–358

26. Shapeero LG, Vanel D (1999) MR imaging in the follow-up evaluation of aggressive soft tissue tumors. Semin Musculoskelet Radiol 3(2):197–206

27. Shapeero LG, Vanel D, Verstraete KL, Bloem JL (1999) Dynamic contrast-enhanced MR imaging for soft tissue sarcomas. Semin Musculoskelet Radiol 3(2):101–114

28. Johnson GR, Zhuang H, Khan J et al (2003) Roles of positron emission tomography with fluorine-18-deoxyglucose in the detection of local recurrent and distant metastatic sarcoma. Clin Nucl Med 28(10):815–820

29. Wahl RL, Jacene H, Kasamon Y, Lodge MA (2009) From RECIST to PERCIST: evolving considerations for PET response criteria in solid tumors. J Nucl Med 50(Suppl 1):122S–150S

Current Principles of Surgical Management of Retroperitoneal Sarcomas

5

Marco Fiore and Sergio Sandrucci

5.1 Introduction: a Shift from Simple Resection to Liberal Multivisceral Resection

Complete surgical resection is the mainstay of treatment for localized retroperitoneal sarcoma (RPS). The rate of complete resection has improved over the years and is close to 95% in most recent published series, but local failure still represents a challenge in the treatment of this disease [1–6]. In order to improve local control and potentially overall survival, an extended surgical approach (en bloc tumor resection with adherent organs and structures, even if not overtly infiltrated) has been advocated for RPS to achieve macroscopically complete tumor resection and minimize microscopically positive margins [7]. The feasibility and safety of extended resection at experienced centers have been reported, showing a postoperative morbidity rate of 18% and a mortality rate of 3% [8]. Also, long-term morbidity has been described as mild, except in cases of femoral nerve resection [9]. Extended resection also showed an overall survival (OS) advantage, with an estimated gain of 18% at 5 years, particularly in low and intermediate grade tumors [10].

5.2 Survival Advantage in Recent Series

The advantage of extended resection has also been supported in the study run by the Trans-Atlantic Retroperitoneal Sarcoma Working Group (TARPSWG) that recently analyzed the largest available series of RPS patients operated on

M. Fiore (✉)
Sarcoma Service, Department of Surgery, Fondazione IRCCS Istituto Nazionale dei Tumori
Milan, Italy
e-mail: marco.fiore@istitutotumori.mi.it

V. Quagliuolo, A. Gronchi (Eds), *Current Treatment of Retroperitoneal Sarcomas,*
Updates in Surgery
DOI: 10.1007/978-88-470-3980-3_5, © Springer-Verlag Italia 2019

at eight major European and North American referral centers in the modern era
[11]. Five- and 10-year OS rates were 67% and 46%, local recurrences were
26% and 35%, and distant metastases were 21% and 22%, respectively. The
extended surgical approach consisted of resection of the ipsilateral kidney in
55% of cases, left/right colon in 33% and 25% of cases, psoas muscle in 27%,
spleen/distal pancreas in 16% and 12%, diaphragm in 13%, abdominal wall
in 12%, iliac vein and/or inferior vena cava (IVC) in 10%. Overall, complete
resection was obtained in 95% and tumor rupture was described in 6% of
patients. When compared with the SEER (Surveillance, Epidemiology, and End
Results) population-based study published in 2009 [12], a 20% difference in OS
until the 10-year time point was shown.

5.3   Surgical Planning

Although the European Society for Medical Oncology (ESMO) guidelines
have recognized this approach as the best therapeutic option for primary RPS
[7], the optimal extent of resection for the single patient is far from standard.
Specifically, whether a single organ has to be resected systematically or only
if directly invaded by the tumor mass is still hard to define. Nonetheless, a
large amount of information is offered for individualized decision-making and
many efforts have been made by experts to define a standard surgical procedure
[13–15]. A critical approach should be driven by anatomic and histologic
considerations, as well as the expected morbidity due to each resected organ [16,
17]. A key point in decision-making should be the rate of microscopic infiltration
of surrounding organs by RPS, which has been described both in the form of
parenchymal invasion as well as of pericapsular/perivisceral invasion in up to
60% of resected organs, with different patterns in different histologies [18–21].
A second key point is the different pattern of relapse of the single histologic
type, as discussed later. A group of experts has recently drawn recommendations
on the extent of surgery, based on existing data from retrospective analyses
of prospectively maintained datasets and, where available, prospective studies
[14]. The principles of recommended practice from diagnosis to follow-up
evaluation are briefly recalled in Table 5.1.

5.3.1   Retroperitoneum Boundaries and Barriers

The retroperitoneum includes multiple vital structures and it extends from the
diaphragm superiorly to the pelvic brim inferiorly. The boundaries are represented by the following structures; anteriorly, the peritoneum, ipsilateral colon
and mesocolon, pancreas, duodenum, spleen, liver and stomach; laterally, the

transversalis fascia with the muscular wall; posteriorly, the quadratus lumbo-rum, psoas, and iliac muscles; medially, the spine, IVC, and aorta; superiorly, the liver and diaphragm.

While the retroperitoneum is not a true anatomic compartment, from the surgical oncologist's standpoint, few anatomic structures that may well work as natural barriers to tumor spread are recognizable: muscle sheaths posteriorly, adventitia of great vessels medially and the peritoneum itself anteriorly can be considered as barriers. Surgical dissection over these barriers should be performed in order to minimize marginality of the overall procedure, in a manner that closely resembles the principles of compartmental resection in the extremities [16]. Where a barrier is not found, the adequacy of margins may be ameliorated by an organ itself, as happens on the anterior part of the tumor when the colon, mesocolon and distal pancreas are resected. Specific knowledge of the retroperitoneal space is important also to minimize the risk of intra- and perioperative morbidity, namely massive bleeding.

5.3.2   Extension of Resection

Once an extended multivisceral resection is planned, preservation of specific organs should be considered on an individualized basis and mandates specific expertise [19]. Appropriate decisions should be ruled out given the overall tumor extent/expected biology and given the individual patient's characteristics. A balance between surgical margins adequacy and expected morbidity is required for each patient. In general, the most common procedures will include en bloc resection of the ipsilateral colon, kidney, adrenal, and psoas muscle; in up to 40% of left-sided RPS distal pancreas and spleen may be necessary, while in only 4–5% of right-sided RPS a pancreaticoduodenectomy is required. Vascular resections are required in up to 12% of cases, predominantly leiomyosarcomas, often originating from major veins. Spine and pelvic bone resection are very rarely needed [16].

5.3.3   Surgical Steps for Standard Resection

The most common surgical access is a midline incision. For better exposure, transverse or oblique extension, or thoracoabdominal incision may be performed, since vascular control is critical. The first step is coloepiploic separation. Then the transverse colon is divided. For right-sided RPS, the distal ileum is divided, and the right colic and ileocolic vessels are divided close to the superior mesenteric vessels. Complete access to the IVC is obtained by a generous Kocher maneuver. Every care should be taken to dissect the duodenum/head of the pancreas from the superomedial aspect of the tumor on a plane very close to the duodenal wall. Occasionally resection of the lateral aspect of

Table 5.1 Consensus Statements from the Trans-Atlantic Retroperitoneal Sarcoma Working Group (extract) [14]

Main statement	RPS is best managed by an experienced multidisciplinary team in specialized referral centers.	IV A
Staging/Preoperative	Standard staging is CT scan of the chest/abdomen/pelvis with IV contrast.	V A
	Functional assessment of the contralateral kidney is necessary and may be achieved using CT with IV contrast or differential renal scanning	V A
	Image-guided percutaneous coaxial core needle biopsy (14 or 16 gauge) is strongly recommended.	IV A
	Risk of needle track seeding is minimal and should not be a reason to avoid a biopsy.	IV A
	Laparotomy and open biopsy of suspected RPS should be avoided.	V E
Primary surgical approach	The best chance of resection with curative intent is at the time of primary presentation.	III A
	Biologic behavior, response to treatment, and clinical outcomes vary by histologic subtype. Management plan and plan for resection should be developed accordingly.	III A
	Complete gross resection is the cornerstone of management.	IIIA
	The aim of surgery should be to achieve macroscopically complete resection, with a single specimen encompassing the tumor and involved contiguous organs, and to minimize positive margins. The best approach is resecting the tumor en bloc with adherent structures even if not overtly infiltrated.	III A
	Preservation of specific organs should be considered on an individualized basis and mandates specific expertise in the disease.	V A
	Technical expertise in multiple sites throughout the abdominal and pelvic cavity is required. Single organ or site expertise is not sufficient.	V A
	Surgical expertise in RPS resection requires specific anatomic knowledge of the RP space to minimize the risk of morbidity.	V A
	Grossly incomplete resection of RPS is of questionable benefit and potentially harmful. It has to be avoided by informed imaging review, thoughtful planning, and referral to another center if appropriate.	III A
	Advanced postoperative monitoring environment is appropriate.	V A
	Immediate or delayed serious life-threatening complications can develop after RPS resection.	V A
	LPS is the most common RPS subtype: its main site of recurrence is intra-abdominal/loco-regional in the erstwhile retroperitoneum.	III A
	Low-grade LPS intraoperatively appears similar to normal fat, and frozen section evaluation is not helpful. The extent of resection in LPS should be guided by asymmetry shown on CT scan, functional anatomy, and experience with patterns of recurrence. Complete resection of all RP fatty tissue is ideal.	III A

Continue →

Adjuvant/neoadjuvant therapies	Although no randomized trials are available, neoadjuvant therapy (chemotherapy; chemotherapy plus hyperthermia; external beam RT; RT plus chemotherapy) is safe for well-selected patients and may be considered by a multidisciplinary sarcoma board. This is particularly relevant in cases of unresectable/borderline resectable RPS and for sensitive histologies.	IV C V C
	Intraoperative RT, postoperative/adjuvant external beam RT and brachytherapy are of no study-proven value and may be associated with significant short- and long-term toxicities.	IV E
	Postoperative/adjuvant chemotherapy is of no study-proven value.	I E
Follow-up evaluation	Risk of recurrence after grossly complete resection of RPS does not plateau, even after 15 to 20 years. Patients should be followed indefinitely.	III A
	Median time to recurrence of high-grade RPS is less than 5 years after definitive treatment.	III A

CT, computed tomography; *LPS*, liposarcoma; *RP*, retroperitoneal; *RPS*, retroperitoneal sarcoma; *RT*, radiation therapy.

Level of evidence
I   Evidence from at least one large randomized control trial of good methodological quality (low potential for bias) or meta-analyses of well-conducted randomized trials without heterogeneity;
III Prospective cohort studies;
IV Retrospective cohort studies or case–control studies;
V   Studies without control group, case reports, experts opinions.

Grade of Recommendation
A   Strong evidence for efficacy with a substantial clinical benefit, strongly recommended;
C   Insufficient evidence for efficacy or benefit does not outweigh the risk or the disadvantages (adverse events, costs), optional
E   Strong evidence against efficacy or for adverse outcome, never recommended.

the duodenum may be required and a primary suture or a jejunal patch is then performed to repair it. The right liver lobe is often simply raised. Occasionally, a more extended mobilization may be required. If not directly invaded though, liver resection is never indicated, while a subcapsular dissection of the inferior and posterior surface may be more often needed. In these situations, liver vascular control is mandatory. For left-sided RPS, the inferior mesenteric vein is ligated at the inferior edge of the pancreas. The inferior mesenteric artery is ligated and the sigmoid colon is divided at the rectosigmoid junction. The mesocolon is then detached from the great vessels. For left RPS confined below the transverse mesocolon, the distal pancreas and spleen are detached from the top of the tumor. For those extending into the upper left retroperitoneum, the distal pancreas is also divided, and the splenic artery and vein ligated. The spleen is mobilized en bloc with the upper portion of the tumor. The great vessels are accessed and prepared by subadventitial dissection from the iliac vessels up to the diaphragmatic hiatus. Collateral branches from the aorta and cava are ligated and divided, including renal, gonadal, and adrenal vessels. The

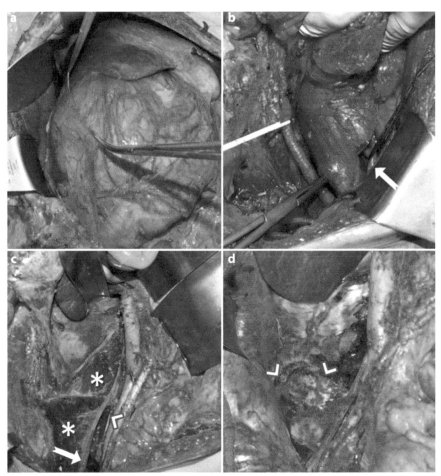

Fig. 5.1 a Approach to the lateral side of retroperitoneal sarcoma is performed by resection of the parietal peritoneum, retroperitoneal dissection will be then conducted up to the psoas muscle on the back of the tumor. **b** Dissection of the great vessels is conducted from the iliac vessel under the adventitia, the psoas muscle is divided over the inguinal ligament, then the femoral nerve is found posteriorly to its lateral edge (*arrow*). **c** After complete psoas muscle resection, the iliac and quadratus lumborum muscles (*asterisks*), the femoral nerve (*arrow*) and obturator nerve (*arrowhead*) are preserved on the back. **d** If directly infiltrated, also the iliac and quadratus lumborum muscles may be resected; this is best obtained en bloc with iliac crest resection (*arrowheads*)

adrenal gland is kept on the specimen to accomplish complete clearance of the upper retroperitoneal space. On the external side, the parietal wall is incised and the peritoneum, or the peritoneum and the internal layer of abdominal side wall are left on the tumor side (Fig. 5.1a). The retroperitoneal dissection should reach the psoas muscle medially. The femoral nerve is identified just above the inguinal ligament after the fascia of the psoas muscle is opened. Then this fascia is detached from the vertebrae and is left on the back side of the tumor. When the psoas is involved it is resected from just superior to the inguinal ligament (Fig. 5.1b) and detached from the spine. Diaphragmatic peritoneum is detached and left on the top of the tumor. The tumor is finally removed en bloc with the kidney, adrenal, ipsilateral colon, and mesocolon in front; aponeurosis of psoas or the whole psoas at the back; peritoneum of the abdominal wall laterally and inferiorly; and peritoneum of diaphragm at the top [13].

5.3.4   Psoas Muscle and Retroperitoneal Nerves

Complete or partial resection of the psoas muscle is needed in roughly 30% of cases (Fig. 5.1c) [11]. Therefore, appropriate knowledge of retroperitoneal musculoskeletal anatomy is warranted. Lumbar arteries and veins, as well as the L2-L4 roots of the femoral and obturator nerves lie behind the fibers of the psoas muscle. The femoral nerve is the major motor nerve in the retroperitoneum and it is found at the posterior and lateral aspect of the psoas muscle, proximally to the inguinal ligament. Patients who undergo complete or partial psoas muscle resection showed a significantly worse lower limb functional score than those who did not [9]. This is obviously even more evident in the case of resection of the femoral nerve. In front of the psoas muscle, the genitofemoral nerve is found, which usually needs to be divided even in cases of partial resection of the psoas or its fascia, resulting in a numbness of the anterior thigh. Other retroperitoneal nerves are found that deserve care during surgery (Fig. 5.2). The

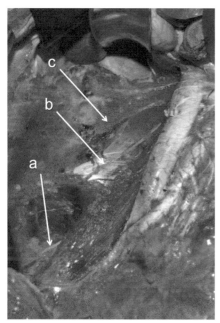

Fig. 5.2 Retroperitoneal sensory nerves: lateral femoral cutaneous nerve (**a**), ilioinguinal nerve (**b**), iliohypogastric nerve (also motor fibers for abdominal side wall) (**c**)

lateral femoral cutaneous and the ilioinguinal are both sensory nerves affecting sensitivity, while the iliohypogastric nerve has also a motor component for the muscles of the lateral abdominal wall. In case the iliohypogastric nerve is divided, it results in a *relaxatio* of the ipsilateral abdominal wall. Sensory disorders of the thigh, groin or genital region have been reported in the long term after surgery by 76% of patients [9].

5.3.5   Other Musculoskeletal Surgical Procedures

According to anatomic presentation of RPS, other musculoskeletal resections may be required. Often the diaphragm has to be partially resected either because directly infiltrated, or in order to safely handle bulky masses occupying the upper abdominal quadrants avoiding tumor rupture. The quadratus lumborum and muscles of the anterior and lateral abdominal wall may also be resected (Fig. 5.3). A mesh repair is often needed in these cases. In cases of RPS extension through the groin, a resection of the psoas muscle up to the insertion on the lesser trochanter is needed. This is better obtained by an abdominoinguinal incision. In the case of inguinal ligament division or inguinal canal resection, a mesh repair will be required to avoid crural herniation (Fig. 5.3). Also bone resections are sometimes needed. The iliac crest, iliac muscle with or without iliac wing may be resected en bloc with the quadratus lumborum (Fig. 5.1d). On the medial aspect of the tumor, transverse pedicles of the vertebrae may need to be resected. Rarely, if tumor invasion within the vertebral foramen is documented, a spine resection (hemivertebral resection) may be indicated.

5.4   Tailoring the Approach to Histology Subtype

Histologic subtype is one of the major determinants for deciding the extent of surgery. Liposarcomas are ill-defined masses, without a clear separation between the well-differentiated component of the tumor and the normal retroperitoneal fat; it has predominantly a risk of local recurrence and 75% of the patients who die do so for inoperable locoregional recurrences. High grade dedifferentiated liposarcomas also have a high metastatic risk, but they share the locoregional characteristics of all other liposarcomas. At the other end of the spectrum, leiomyosarcoma shows the highest rate of distant metastases with very low risk of local recurrence. In addition, leiomyosarcomas tend to have a well-defined macroscopic appearance, making it easier to separate the tumor form adjacent uninvolved structures, without compromising the quality of surgical margins. Likewise, solitary fibrous tumors have a well-defined appearance, with both limited local recurrence and distant metastatic risks. Malignant peripheral

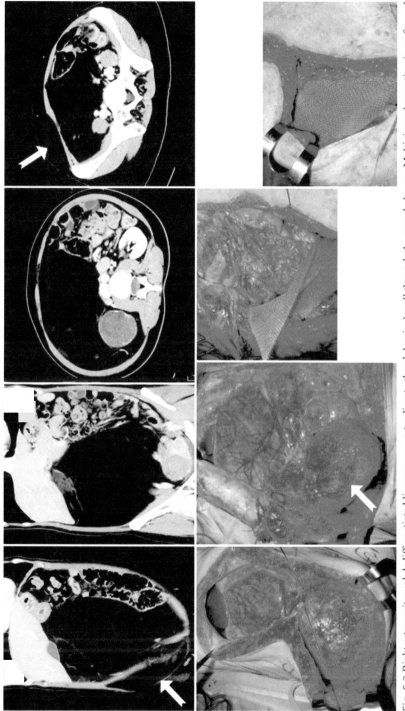

Fig. 5.3 Right retroperitoneal dedifferentiated liposarcoma extending to the abdominal wall through the muscle layers. Multivisceral resection is performed en bloc with anterolateral abdominal wall and inguinal ligament. Parietal defect and inguinal ligament are repaired by polypropylene mesh interposition. The greater omentum is placed behind the mesh to cover the small bowel

nerve sheath tumors (MPNST) usually arise from the femoral nerve and are located in the context of the psoas muscle. A specific approach for this disease is then warranted [11, 22]. For these reason, in a simplistic manner, we suggest systematically resecting the surrounding organs in liposarcoma variants, while approaching leiomyosarcoma, solitary fibrous tumor and MPNST in a more conservative manner. Rarer histologic subtypes require even more specific expert knowledge in order to assure the best multidisciplinary approach.

5.4.1 Vascular Retroperitoneal Sarcoma

Retroperitoneal sarcomas of vascular origin are a rare subset of RPS worthy of mention. They primarily arise from a vein, the IVC being the most frequent, followed by the renal vein, iliac vein, splenic vein, gonadal vein, and superior mesenteric vein [23–25]. They are predominately leiomyosarcomas [26]. The surgical approach will necessarily require resection of the vessel of origin.

5.5   The Case of Pelvic Sarcomas

While in cases of bulky masses RPS commonly extend to the pelvis, in approximately 18% of cases the tumor is exclusively located within the pelvic region [5]. Uterine sarcomas and pediatric rhabdomyosarcomas are also pelvic tumors, but are not included in this review and deserve a different approach. The most frequent pelvic RPS are leiomyosarcomas, which often originate directly from pelvic viscera (bladder, prostate, seminal vesicles); however, also nerve sheath tumors (both schwannomas and MPNST), aggressive angiomyxomas and solitary fibrous tumors are not infrequent. A peculiar presentation of pelvic RPS is the one of well-differentiated liposarcoma that may herniate through the obturator or sciatic notch (dumbbell tumors) [27]. Pelvic RPS present unique challenges given the narrow anatomic confines of the bony pelvis and the major functional deficits that may result from their resection in the event that pelvic organs and structures need to be resected. For these reasons, pelvic sarcomas are best managed at high-volume centers. In fact, a highly individualized multidisciplinary treatment is paramount, and it has to be primarily based on specific histology.

5.6   Conclusions

Current principles for adequate surgical resection of primary RPS include a variety of technical skills that encompass usual single organ-oriented procedures.

RPS are a rare and complex disease, and extensive knowledge of sarcoma biology and behavior of histologic subtypes is overriding to establish the adequate extent of surgery. Primary RPS are best managed by extensive resection of the tumor en bloc with surrounding structures, even if not grossly infiltrated. A multidisciplinary approach and referral to experienced centers is required to guarantee the best chance of cure of primary RPS.

References

1. Lewis JJ, Leung D, Woodruff JM, Brennan MF (1998) Retroperitoneal soft-tissue sarcoma: analysis of 500 patients treated and followed at a single institution. Ann Surg 228(3): 355–365
2. Keung EZ, Hornick JL, Bertagnolli MM et al (2014) Predictors of outcomes in patients with primary retroperitoneal dedifferentiated liposarcoma undergoing surgery. J Am Coll Surg 218(2):206–217
3. Strauss DC, Hayes AJ, Thway K et al (2010) Surgical management of primary retroperitoneal sarcoma. Br J Surg 97(5):698–706
4. Bonvalot S, Rivoire M, Castaing M et al (2009) Primary retroperitoneal sarcomas: a multivariate analysis of surgical factors associated with local control. J Clin Oncol 27(1):31–37
5. Gronchi A, Lo Vullo S, Fiore M et al (2009) Aggressive surgical policies in a retrospectively reviewed single-institution case series of retroperitoneal soft tissue sarcoma patients. J Clin Oncol 27(1):24–30
6. Gronchi A, Miceli R, Allard MA et al (2015) Personalizing the approach to retroperitoneal soft tissue sarcoma: histology-specific patterns of failure and postrelapse outcome after primary extended resection. Ann Surg Oncol 22(5):1447–1454
7. Casali PG, Abecassis N, Bauer S et al (2018) Soft tissue and visceral sarcomas: ESMO-EURACAN Clinical Practice Guidelines for diagnosis, treatment and follow-up. Ann Oncol [Epub ahead of print] doi:10.1093/annonc/mdy096
8. Berselli M, Coppola S, Colombo C et al (2011) Morbidity of left pancreatectomy when associated with multivisceral resection for abdominal mesenchymal neoplasms. JOP 12(2):138–144
9. Callegaro D, Miceli R, Brunelli C et al (2015) Long-term morbidity after multivisceral resection for retroperitoneal sarcoma. Br J Surg 102(9):1079–1087
10. Gronchi A, Miceli R, Colombo C et al (2012) Frontline extended surgery is associated with improved survival in retroperitoneal low- to intermediate-grade soft tissue sarcomas. Ann Oncol 23(4):1067–1073
11. Gronchi A, Strauss DC, Miceli R et al (2016) Variability in patterns of recurrence after resection of primary retroperitoneal sarcoma (RPS): a report on 1007 patients from the Multi-institutional Collaborative RPS Working Group. Ann Surg 263(5):1002–1009
12. Nathan H, Raut CP, Thornton K et al (2009) Predictors of survival after resection of retroperitoneal sarcoma: a population-based analysis and critical appraisal of the AJCC staging system. Ann Surg 250(6):970–976
13. Bonvalot S, Raut CP, Pollock RE et al (2012) Technical considerations in surgery for retroperitoneal sarcomas: position paper from E-Surge, a master class in sarcoma surgery, and EORTC-STBSG. Ann Surg Oncol 19(9):2981–2991
14. Trans-Atlantic RPS Working Group (2015) Management of primary retroperitoneal sarcoma (RPS) in the adult: a consensus approach from the Trans-Atlantic RPS Working Group. Ann Surg Oncol 22(1):256–263

15. Fairweather M, Gonzalez RJ, Strauss D, Raut CP (2018) Current principles of surgery for retroperitoneal sarcomas. J Surg Oncol 117(1):33–41
16. Callegaro D, Fiore M, Gronchi A (2015) Personalizing surgical margins in retroperitoneal sarcomas. Expert Rev Anticancer Ther 15(5):553–567
17. MacNeill AJ, Fiore M (2018) Surgical morbidity in retroperitoneal sarcoma resection. J Surg Oncol 117(1):56–61
18. Mussi C, Colombo P, Bertuzzi A et al (2011) Retroperitoneal sarcoma: is it time to change the surgical policy? Ann Surg Oncol 18(8):2136–2142
19. Strauss DC, Renne SL, Gronchi A (2018) Adjacent, adherent, invaded: a spectrum of biologic aggressiveness rather than a rationale for selecting organ resection in surgery of primary retroperitoneal sarcomas. Ann Surg Oncol 25(1):13–16
20. Renne SL, Tagliabue M, Pasquali S et al (2017) Prognostic value of microscopic evaluation of organ infiltration and visceral resection margins (VRM) in patients with retroperitoneal sarcomas (RPS). JCO 35(15 Suppl):11074–11074
21. Fairweather M, Wang J, Jo VY et al (2018) Surgical management of primary retroperitoneal sarcomas: rationale for selective organ resection. Ann Surg Oncol 25(1):98–106
22. Gronchi A, Collini P, Miceli R et al (2015) Myogenic differentiation and histologic grading are major prognostic determinants in retroperitoneal liposarcoma. Am J Surg Pathol 39(3):383–393
23. Fiore M, Colombo C, Locati P et al (2012) Surgical technique, morbidity, and outcome of primary retroperitoneal sarcoma involving inferior vena cava. Ann Surg Oncol 19(2):511–518
24. Radaelli S, Fiore M, Colombo C et al (2016) Vascular resection en-bloc with tumor removal and graft reconstruction is safe and effective in soft tissue sarcoma (STS) of the extremities and retroperitoneum. Surg Oncol 25(3):125–131
25. Fiore M, Radaelli S, Gronchi A (2017) Retroperitoneal sarcoma involving the vena cava. In: Azoulay D, Lim C, Salloum C (eds) Surgery of the inferior vena cava. Springer International Publishing, pp 61–74
26. Ito H, Hornick JL, Bertagnolli MM et al (2007) Leiomyosarcoma of the inferior vena cava: survival after aggressive management. Ann Surg Oncol 14(12):3534–3541
27. Mullen JT, van Houdt W (2018) Soft tissue tumors of the pelvis: technical and histological considerations. J Surg Oncol 117(1):48–55

Managing Early and Late Postoperative Complications

6

Stefano Radaelli and Sergio Valeri

6.1.   Background

Surgery is the cornerstone of treatment for retroperitoneal sarcoma (RPS). Due to the remarkable size these tumors can reach at the diagnosis and the potential involvement of surrounding organs, surgery may require extended visceral resections in order to provide the best chance of local control. A correct therapeutic plan should therefore consider the complexity of surgery in the face of possible perioperative complications. Given the rarity of the disease and the heterogeneity of the treatment strategies, only few groups have described early and late outcomes after RPS resection. Despite these limitations, a detailed overview of short- and long-term morbidity and of the related management will be discussed in the following paragraphs.

6.2   Extent of Surgery and Postoperative Morbidity

The surgical approach to RPS has changed completely over the last ten years, shifting toward a liberal en bloc resection of tumor-adherent organs.

Although the survival benefit from a frontline extended surgical approach was widely proved [1–4], a heated debate was focused on the potential risk of increased postoperative complications [5–6]. This question was addressed in a recent retrospective trial by the Trans-Atlantic Retroperitoneal Sarcoma Working Group (TARPSWG), an international collaboration of the major

S. Radaelli (✉)
Sarcoma Service, Department of Surgery, Fondazione IRCCS Istituto Nazionale dei Tumori
Milan, Italy
e-mail: stefano.radaelli@istitutotumori.mi.it

V. Quagliuolo, A. Gronchi (Eds), *Current Treatment of Retroperitoneal Sarcomas,*
Updates in Surgery
DOI: 10.1007/978-88-470-3980-3_6, © Springer-Verlag Italia 2019

sarcoma referral centers worldwide. Data of 1007 patients affected by primary and localized RPS treated from 2002 to 2011 in eight specialist sarcoma institutions were merged and analyzed. The 30-day mortality rate in this series was 1.8%, with 16.4% of patients suffering a major complication (Clavien-Dindo ≥3) and 10.5% requiring reoperation. The most common adverse events were bleeding/hematoma (2.9%) and gastrointestinal anastomotic leak (2.6%).

Interestingly, the pattern of complications was categorized not only by the number of organs resected but also according to a specific resected organ score, proving that resection of some organs or structures entails a higher risk of morbidity than others. The weighted resected organ score was therefore a relevant prognosticator for morbidity along with elderly age (>65 years) and transfusion requirements. The most critical patterns of resection associated with a higher risk of major adverse events were: pancreaticoduodenectomy, vascular resection, and the simultaneous resection of colon, kidney, spleen, and pancreas. Conversely, perioperative administration of chemo-radiation therapy was not related to worse postoperative morbidity. Importantly, no association between surgical morbidity and local or distant failure was documented, suggesting that the quality of postoperative recovery did not correlate with the oncologic outcome [7].

Some years ago, the French and Italian sarcoma centers published their own initial series of frontline extended resections, reporting their combined morbidity rate to prove the feasibility and safety of their novel surgical approach. In this cohort of primary RPS, 30-day mortality was 3%, severe complications (CTCAE ≥3) occurred in 18%, and 12% required a second operation. Most common complications were gastrointestinal anastomotic leak (5.2%), abscess (4%), and bleeding (2.4%). Postoperative morbidity increased significantly with resection of more than three organs (HR 2.75, 95% CI, 1.32–5.74; p=0.007). Resection of stomach, small bowel (mainly duodenum), and major vessels was also associated with a higher incidence of adverse events [4].

Further results on the short-term postoperative outcome have been also separately provided by several sarcoma tertiary centers across the world. Unfortunately, these data are not completely homogenous since a liberal multivisceral surgical approach was not routinely performed.

In the decade between 2005 and 2014, 362 resections for primary RPS were performed at the Royal Marsden Hospital. Only 81% of patients underwent multivisceral resections and this might explain the more favorable outcome of this series when compared to earlier experience with radical resection. Mortality rates at 30, 60, and 90 days were 1.4%, 1.9%, and 3.0%, respectively; severe morbidity (Clavien-Dindo ≥3) rate was 9%; reoperation rate was 7.5% [8].

Similar results were also reported in three smaller series of patients treated with a more conservative approach in the pre-radical resection era. Ninety-seven patients underwent surgery for primary RPS at the Mayo Clinic between 1983 and 1995. Only 22.7% of them had more than one organ resected. In-hospital mortality was 2%, major complications occurred in 8%, and 6% underwent reoperation [9]. From the Dutch National Database, a group of 143 patients surgically treated for primary RPS between 1989 and 1994 was retrieved and analyzed. Operative details are not reported but macroscopic complete resection was achieved in only 63% of patients, as compared to 93% in the French-Italian series and 95% in the TARPSWG experience. Thirty-day mortality in the Dutch population study was 4% [10].

A single-center experience from Heidelberg reported on 110 patients operated on for RPS between 1988 and 2002. This series counted both primary (n=71) and recurrent (n=39) RPS. Extent of surgery is not reported but complete resection was achieved in 70.4% of primary RPS and 61.5% of recurrent tumors. Mortality at 30 days was 6.4%, with no significant difference between primary RPS and recurrent disease (7.0% vs. 5.1%, $p=1.0$). The overall morbidity rate was 26%, again with no remarkable difference between resection for primary vs. recurrent RPS (24% vs. 31%, $p=0.41$) [11].

The sizeable Memorial Sloan Kettering Cancer Center database included 278 patients who underwent surgery for primary RPS between 1982 and 1997, of whom 77% had at least one organ resected. Mortality in this population was 4% at 30 days [12].

A peculiar view on RPS treatment was given by the MD Anderson Cancer Center, which tailored a specific surgical approach based on tumor histology. From 1996 to 2007, 135 patients affected by both primary and recurrent retroperitoneal liposarcoma were surgically treated, adopting a more conservative approach for well-differentiated liposarcoma (WDLPS), while a liberal en bloc resection was preferred for dedifferentiated liposarcoma (DDLPS). The postoperative complications reflected the two alternative approaches: mortality and morbidity in the WDLPS group was 0% and 15% respectively, compared to 3.9% and 35.1%, respectively, in the DDLPS group [13].

Outside referral centers, RPS are generally treated with a more conservative approach. Tseng et al. reported a series of 156 patients undergoing resection of retroperitoneal tumors in 255 hospitals including both community and university centers. Patients were marginally excised in most of the cases, approximately one-third underwent resection of adjacent organs and only a minority were systematically treated with multivisceral resections. In this series of predominantly conservative resections, 30-day mortality was still 1.3%, severe morbidity 22.5%, and the reoperation rate 4.5% [14].

Regarding the wide spectrum of postoperative morbidity (Table 6.1), we want to focus on some peculiar complications which, if misdiagnosed, may worsen patients' clinical condition and prolong their hospitalization.

One of the most challenging aspects is the diagnosis and treatment of pancreatic fistula (output via an operatively placed drain – or subsequently placed percutaneous drain – of any measurable volume of drain fluid on or after postoperative day 3, with an amylase content greater than 3 times the upper normal

Table 6.1 Largest retroperitoneal sarcoma series reporting postoperative morbidity rates

Author	n. of patients	Median FU (months)	% events (III-IV)	% death (30 days)	% bleeding	% anastomotic leak	% pancreatic leak
Strauss DC, 2010 [15]	200	29	12	3	3	-	-
Bonvalot S, 2010 [4]	249	37	18	3	2.4	5.2	-
Berselli M, 2011* [16]	57	32	35.1	3.5	3.5	3.5	12.3
Nussbaum DP, 2014[17]	216	-	27.3	2.7	14.8	-	-
Bartlett EK, 2014 [18]	696	-	30	1	13	-	-
Kelly KJ, 2015 [19]	204	39	6.3	0	1.9	1.9	-
Smith HG, 2015 [8]	362	26	8.8	1.4	-	2.2	17
Pasquali S, 2015 [20]	69	31	23	0	2.9	5.8	-
MacNeill AJ, 2017 [7]	1007	58	16.4	1.8	2.9	2.6	<1

* Series of retroperitoneal sarcoma (45 patients) and gastrointestinal stromal tumor (12 patients).

serum value, according to the classification of the International Study Group of Pancreatic Fistula [ISGPF] classification) following distal pancreatectomy as part of left RPS resection. The reported rate of pancreatic leakage may vary between below 10% and above 30% when pancreatic resections are carried out at high volume centers for pancreatic disease [21–25]. In the TARPSWG cohort the reported incidence is less than 1%, but that series concerns all the RPS cases with or without pancreatic resection and is therefore not comparable [7].

In 2012 Berselli et al. retrospectively analyzed the postoperative outcome of 57 patients affected by localized left RPS or intra-abdominal gastrointestinal stromal tumors (GIST) treated at the same referral center. The RPS were 79% and the GIST were 21%. The aim of the study was to evaluate the morbidity of distal pancreatectomy when associated with multivisceral resection for abdominal mesenchymal neoplasms. Sectioning of the pancreas was performed in all cases but one using a mechanical stapler. Macroscopic complete resection was achieved in all patients but three (5%). Pancreatic involvement was documented at pathology in 26 cases (46%). Twenty patients (35%) suffered from surgical complication and seven patients (12%) developed a postoperative pancreatic fistula (one grade A, five grade B, and one grade C) with two of them requiring a second operation. The postoperative mortality rate was 3.5%: two patients died and during their complex clinical course, developed a pancreatic leakage, although it was not ascribed as the ultimate cause of death. Apparently preoperative chemo-radiation therapy was not associated with a higher risk of pancreatic fistula: in fact, only one patient developing a postoperative pancreatic leakage underwent neoadjuvant treatments [16].

A similar rate of pancreatic leakage was reported also at the Royal Marsden Hospital. Among 362 patients undergoing surgery for RPS, 292 received a multivisceral resection, and left pancreatectomy was performed in 60 patients. Eight of them (17%) developed a pancreatic fistula with a median time of recovery of 18 days. Only two patients underwent percutaneous drainage [8].

The treatment approach of the pancreatic fistula normally reflects its clinical relevance:

- *Grade A* is treated conservatively. Amylase levels are routinely measured in the drain tubes on alternative days and the drain can be removed according to the quality (absence of pancreatic component) and quantity (less than 50 mL per day) of the output.
- *Grade B* normally requires antibiotic treatment and octreotide. In the presence of a large or symptomatic collection a percutaneous drainage should be performed (Fig. 6.1) and if not feasible a transgastric approach may be considered. The drain removal will follow the same criteria for the Grade A fistula.
- *Grade C* has to be considered a serious clinical event and needs to be properly treated even with reintervention if the more conservative treatments have failed.

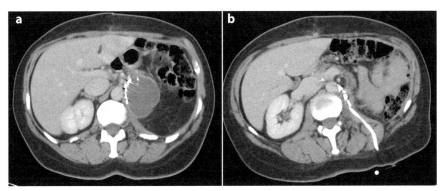

Fig. 6.1 a Left retroperitoneal pancreatic fluid collection following multivisceral en bloc retroperitoneal sarcoma resection with distal pancreatectomy. **b** Collection resolution after percutaneous drainage

A systematic review from Knaebel et al. did not draw any conclusion regarding the optimal surgical technique for pancreatic stump closure aiming to decrease the incidence of pancreatic leak; however, they described a trend in favor of the stapling technique [26]. Furthermore, no differences in the overall complication rate were found by comparing two groups of patients undergoing distal pancreatectomy straightforwardly or as part of multivisceral resection for a contiguous tumor [27].

Late symptoms from pancreatic leakage may include also delayed gastric emptying (Fig. 6.2). This complication may often be related to the presence of a large left retroperitoneal collection right behind the posterior gastric wall. The pancreatic fluid can displace the stomach also promoting a local inflammatory condition which may be considered one of the causes of gastroparesis. In addition, the extended retroperitoneal dissection, which may entail sacrifice of the gastric branches of the vagus nerve and the empty space generated by the excision of the retroperitoneal mass en bloc with distal pancreas and spleen, responsible for the posterior displacement of the stomach, may certainly affect gastric motility.

Treatment of delayed gastric emptying depends on the impact on patient quality of life. Save in exceptional cases, recovery occurs fast and never requires surgical re-intervention. In the presence of a large fluid retroperitoneal collection maintaining the gastroparesis, a percutaneous evacuative puncture or the insertion of a temporary drain is always recommended. Nutritional support with enteral nutrition via a nasogastric feeding tube combined with administration of prokinetic drugs should be always considered in those rare cases of refractory delayed gastric emptying [16, 28].

A particular situation increasing the risk of postoperative morbidity concerns the vascular involvement of the main retroperitoneal vessels in the context of multivisceral RPS resection. Notably, the inferior vena cava (IVC) replacement

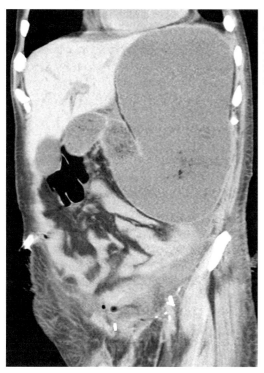

Fig. 6.2 Delayed gastric emptying after left retroperitoneal sarcoma en bloc resection with distal pancreatectomy, splenectomy, nephrectomy, left colonic and psoas muscle resection

is often a technical challenge which may lead to severe postoperative sequelae. The main concern about IVC resection and reconstruction regards the higher risk of bleeding. Although any leakage from venous graft or artificial prosthesis should be prevented, it may seldom occur and if not urgently treated may become fatal. Besides, the stronger anticoagulation medications usually used in the perioperative period affect the risk of bleeding and may lead to developing large retroperitoneal hematoma, which needs to be surgically removed to avoid severe infections.

The development of graft thrombosis may occur in the medium-long term after IVC reconstruction despite ongoing anticoagulant therapy. It does not usually represent a serious adverse event, often being asymptomatic especially in the presence of collaterals. Reconstruction with banked cadaveric homograft instead of synthetic prosthesis is normally associated with a lower rate of complications including vascular thrombosis and therefore its use should be privileged. The caval filter is not required unless there is a free-floating thrombus or anticoagulant treatment has failed [29–32].

Pancreaticoduodenectomy is only occasionally part of the multivisceral resection and does increase the incidence of postoperative morbidity. A recent series of 2068 patients published by the TARPSWG reported only 29 patients

(1.4%) who underwent a Whipple resection. Among them, 45% underwent concomitant IVC resection. Microscopic invasion of duodenum and pancreas were seen in 84% of cases. Postoperatively, 10 patients (34%) had major complications including eight (28%) who developed a clinically-significant pancreatic leak. One postoperative death (3.4%) occurred [33].

6.3   Impact of Radiotherapy on Perioperative Morbidity

Extrapolating data from studies on soft tissue sarcoma of the extremities, the use of pre- or postoperative radiotherapy (RT) to reduce the local recurrence rate has been increasing in the management of RPS in the last decade. The few available results are controversial since, although neoadjuvant RT was associated with 5-year local recurrence free-survival of 91% in the RT group and 65% in the surgery-only group ($p=0.02$), no survival benefit was reported at 5 years (53.2% vs. 54.2%; $p=0.695$) in one of the larger studies investigating the effectiveness of RT in RPS [19].

The STRASS trial – a randomized controlled trial of the EORTC (European Organisation for Research and Treatment of Cancer) – has been designed to try to address this area of persistent clinical equipoise. While the final trial results are still awaited, the safety of preoperative external beam radiotherapy (EBRT) in the treatment of RPS has been validated on interim analysis, without reporting increased adverse events after resection of irradiated RPS [34, 35].

In the same way a recent large analysis supported the safety profile of preoperative RT in RPS. This retrospective review from the National Surgical Quality Improvement Program (NSQIP), between 2005 and 2011, identified 785 patients presenting with RPS, of whom 72 received neoadjuvant RT. After adjusting for confounding variables, all baseline characteristics were highly similar in the two groups (RT+surgery vs. surgery alone) but there were no differences in mortality (1.4 vs. 2.1%, $p=0.71$), major complications (28.2 vs. 25.2%, $p=0.69$), overall complications (35.2 vs. 33.2%, $p=0.83$), early reoperation (5.6 vs. 7.4%, $p=0.81$), or hospitalization (7 vs. 7 days, $p=0.56$) [18]. The limited benefits produced by the use of EBRT, mostly due to the inability of delivering adequate doses on account of the tolerance limits of adjacent viscera, led a group of radiation oncologists to explore the role of intraoperative radiotherapy (IORT) as part of the treatment of RPS.

Two prospective studies showed encouraging results with respect to local control but documented a higher incidence of postoperative morbidity with this technique. Sindelar et al. reported significant rates of radiation-related peripheral neuropathy while Dziewirski et al., administering intraoperative brachytherapy, reported favorable data in terms of local control and overall survival but a 2% rate of early postoperative mortality and a 21.5% reoperation rate [36, 37].

Recently published data from The Johns Hopkins School of Medicine analyzed outcomes in 113 patients with abdominopelvic malignancies, of which 44% were sarcomas, treated with IORT. The majority of RPS were recurrent (68%) and the choice to deliver IORT was carefully considered for those tumors at a higher risk of positive margins after EBRT and attempt at radical resection. A total of 57% of patients experienced postoperative complications although severe postoperative adverse events (Clavien-Dindo ≥3) occurred in 34% of patients without any death observed [38]. Similarly, a clinical phase I/II trial investigating preoperative intensity-modulated radiation therapy (IMRT) and IORT in patients with RPS reported an unplanned interim safety analysis in 2014 documenting severe acute toxicity (grade 3) in four patients (15%) and severe postoperative complications in nine patients (33%), of whom two finally died after multiple re-interventions [39].

Prohibitive toxicities and no disease control benefits were reported also by Smith et al. in the long-term results of a phase II trial of preoperative radiotherapy (45–50 Gray) plus postoperative brachytherapy. Treatment related mortality was 7.5% at 18 months median follow-up, and severe late toxicities persisted in 11% of patients alive beyond this time point. Specifically, duodenal stenosis was a critical complication in patients treated with brachytherapy in the upper abdomen [40].

In all these recent series, the morbidity following neoadjuvant EBRT + IORT is significantly higher if compare to that reported in the TARPSWG experience with radical resection +/− EBRT.

Based on these available data, a consensus document from the TARPSWG stated that neoadjuvant EBRT may be considered in selected patients and according to peculiar anatomical disease presentation. Intraoperative RT might be considered in the presence of a very critical margin of resection, even though in practice the extension of the intraoperative field is inconsistent with a safe treatment, and there is no evidence of effectiveness. Finally, adjuvant RT is discouraged given the excessive morbidity and the inability to achieve a therapeutic dose [41].

6.4 Long-term Morbidity

Sporadic data exist on the long-term morbidity associated with frontline extended resection of RPS; specific sequelae – such as permanent renal failure, neurological impairment or chronic pain – have never been systematically investigated. As a consequence of the survival improvement in RPS (67% at 5 years for all subtypes and more than 80% at 10 years for well-differentiated liposarcoma) the treatment-related long-term disability is becoming a critical concern in patient management [42, 43].

6.4.1 Renal Function Following Nephrectomy

The question whether en bloc nephrectomy should be routinely performed in the context of RPS multivisceral resection has long been debated in the past. Data regarding the neoplastic invasion of the kidney are controversial, with some authors reporting that this happens in a minority of cases and some others documenting rates approximately as high as 80%. Although a frontline extended approach has been confirmed as the mainstay of treatment for RPS by all major international referral centers, little has been published regarding the long-term risk of chronic kidney disease (CKD) in those patients undergoing nephrectomy [44–47].

In 2015 Hull et al. published a retrospective analysis of long-term renal function following RPS resection with en bloc nephrectomy on 54 patients operated on at Massachusetts General Hospital between 1987 and 2013. Median preoperative estimated glomerular filtration rate (eGFR) was 85 mL/min. Post-nephrectomy, median nadir eGFR was 44 mL/min, recovering to 62 mL/min at a median follow-up of 50 months. Of 49 patients with preoperative eGFR ≥60 mL/min (CKD stage 1, 2), 51% maintained eGFR ≥60 mL/min postoperatively, whereas 49% progressed to CKD stage 3 (eGFR 30–59). Independent risk factors for progression of CKD stage were age and preoperative eGFR. Eleven patients died of recurrent disease while no patient developed end-stage renal disease or required dialysis. In this series, seven patients underwent chemotherapy, either in the adjuvant setting or for subsequent recurrence. Among these, five experienced further progression in CKD class after chemotherapy, nevertheless they were able to receive different systemic therapies, including nephrotoxic agents like ifosfamide [48].

Similar results were also described in a more recent study from the Mayo Clinic, which retrospectively reviewed 47 patients operated on for RPS sarcoma between 1999 and 2014. The primary outcome measured was CKD calculated by GFR. Of the 47 patients in their study cohort, GFR decreased by an average of 33.4 mL/min and 34 (72%) patients showed progression of their renal failure. Of these, three (6%) patients progressed to severe renal disease (CKD stage 4 or 5) in their postoperative course with two of them following administration of ifosfamide based chemotherapy as a result of metastatic disease [44].

Analogous data are reported in the Royal Marsden Hospital experience, in which 113 patients who underwent nephrectomy as part of their RPS resection were monitored with a particular focus on their renal function. The median preoperative eGFR of 89.2 mL/min declined to a nadir of 46 mL/min postoperatively but later rebounded to 58.1 mL/min at a median follow-up of 20.2 months; only one patient who received right nephrectomy, IVC resection and left renal vein ligation required temporary dialysis [8].

Renal function after frontline extended resection for RPS was also investigated by the Milan group in a retrospective analysis of 95 long-term survivors. Nephrectomy was performed in 67% of cases. After nephrectomy, plasmatic creatinine level was within 1.5 times the upper reference limit in 91% of patients both at 4 months after surgery and at the survey time point (median 49 months). In multivariable analysis, adjusting for patient, age and baseline levels, creatinine concentration did not significantly differ between patients who underwent nephrectomy and those who did not [43].

6.4.2 Pain, Function, and Quality of Life

Symptoms related to multivisceral retroperitoneal resection are usually heterogenous and may vary from patient to patient reflecting the extension of the surgical approach. However, a comprehensive review of these aspects has never been provided by any of the studies exploring patient outcomes after RPS resection. Novel results have been recently reported by Wong et al. who analyzed the long-term quality of life (QoL) (EORTC-QLQ-C30) in a series of 48 patients treated with neoadjuvant RT and surgery. The number of post-treatment toxicities significantly ($p=0.001$) impacts QoL, especially during the first 36 postoperative months. QoL at 36 months from surgery was better than at diagnosis [49].

In recent years a particular focus on patients' postoperative symptoms and QoL has been promoted by the Italian group in Milan [43]. A sample of 95 patients operated on in the decade 2002–2011 were enrolled in a retrospective study evaluating long-term morbidity after RPS resection. Neurological impairment, pain and QoL were assessed by means of semi-structured interviews. Sensory disorders occurred in 76% of patients after surgery and were persistent in 62% at the survey time (median 49 months after surgery). Psoas muscle resection resulted in a double proportion of patients with sensory disturbances compared to those with only fascia or without psoas resection ($p<0.0001$). Patients undergoing femoral nerve resection and extended psoas resection experienced significant motor disability in the ipsilateral lower limb as assessed by Lower Extremity Function Scale (LEFS). Similarly, lower LEFS scores were reported in patients who experienced severe postoperative adverse events (Clavien-Dindo ≥ 3). Sexual disorders were commonly described, and loss of libido was reported up to one-third of patients. Dyspareunia affected 22% of women while sexual impotence and retrograde ejaculation 27% and 9% of men, respectively. Chronic pain after surgery was investigated using the Brief Pain Inventory (BPI). The legs were the most common site of pain (39%), followed by the abdomen and back (30%). While 39% never experienced pain symptoms, 21% reported mild pain with a score of at least 5. Interference with daily activities was generally infrequent, mostly regarding walking and ability to work, demonstrating that severe pain is seldom a problem in the long-term period. The retrospective nature of this study and the higher proportion of missing data provided limited information regarding patient function and QoL following RPS surgery.

Prospective results have been recently presented by Fiore et al. who recruited 60 primary RPS patients and investigated QoL and pain by means of the EORTC QLQ-C30. The baseline data regarding Global Health Status (GHS) were similar to all cancer patients when adjusted for patients and age. Mild non-specific symptoms such as fatigue, insomnia and urinary discomfort were reported. Pain was documented in 68% of patients at baseline. Limb neuropathy and functional impairment were reported even before surgery in roughly 50% of patients, indicating that they might be partially tumor-related [50].

6.5   Conclusions

A comprehensive analysis of early and late morbidity following RPS resection have never been performed to date. The only available data from limited and retrospective studies report an acceptable rate of postoperative complications while functional outcome and QoL remain poorly understood. Chronic renal failure following en bloc nephrectomy is seldom observed and the plasmatic levels of creatinine remain slightly above the upper level value. Sensory disorders and neurologic dysfunction represent the major concern affecting patients QoL in the long term.

In order to achieve a full understanding of the impact of RPS and its treatment on patient outcomes, detailed data on morbidity and QoL should be prospectively collected by any sarcoma referral center, ideally validating specific tools within the sarcoma community. Patients diagnosed with a RPS must always be referred to specialized sarcoma centers. Simultaneously, the improvement in surgical skills and the continuous advancement in the learning curve should guarantee the highest quality standards in the pre- and postoperative management of patients.

References

1. Bonvalot S, Rivoire M, Castaing M et al (2009) Primary retroperitoneal sarcomas: a multivariate analysis of surgical factors associated with local control. J Clin Oncol 27(1):31–37
2. Gronchi A, Lo Vullo S, Fiore M et al (2009) Aggressive surgical policies in a retrospectively reviewed single-institution case series of retroperitoneal soft tissue sarcoma patients. J Clin Oncol 27(1):24–30
3. Gronchi A, Miceli R, Colombo C et al (2011) Frontline extended surgery is associated with improved survival in retroperitoneal low- to intermediate-grade soft tissue sarcomas. Ann Oncol 23(4):1067–1073

4. Bonvalot S, Miceli R, Berselli M et al (2010) Aggressive surgery in retroperitoneal soft tissue sarcoma carried out at high-volume centers is safe and is associated with improved local control. Ann Surg Oncol 17(6):1507–1514

5. Pisters PWT (2009) Resection of some – but not all – clinically uninvolved adjacent viscera as part of surgery for retroperitoneal soft tissue sarcomas. J Clin Oncol 27(1):6–8

6. Raut CP, Swallow CJ (2010) Are radical compartmental resections for retroperitoneal sarcomas justified? Ann Surg Oncol 17(6):1481–1484

7. MacNeill AJ, Gronchi A, Miceli R et al (2018) Postoperative morbidity after radical resection of primary retroperitoneal sarcoma: a report from the Transatlantic RPS Working Group. Ann Surg 267(5):959–964

8. Smith HG, Panchalingam D, Hannay JAF et al (2015) Outcome following resection of retroperitoneal sarcoma. Br J Surg 102(13):1698–1709

9. Hassan I, Park SZ, Donohue JH et al (2004) Operative management of primary retroperitoneal sarcomas: a reappraisal of an institutional experience. Ann Surg 239(2): 244–250

10. van Dalen T, Plooij JM, Van Coevorden F et al; Dutch Soft Tissue Sarcoma Group (2007) Long-term prognosis of primary retroperitoneal soft tissue sarcoma. Eur J Surg Oncol 33(2):234–238

11. Lehnert T, Cardona S, Hinz U et al (2009) Primary and locally recurrent retroperitoneal soft-tissue sarcoma: local control and survival. Eur J Surg Oncol 35(9):986–993

12. Lewis JJ, Leung D, Woodruff JM, Brennan MF (1998) Retroperitoneal soft-tissue sarcoma: analysis of 500 patients treated and followed at a single institution. Ann Surg 228(3):355–365

13. Lahat G, Anaya DA, Wang X et al (2008) Resectable well-differentiated versus dedifferentiated liposarcomas: two different diseases possibly requiring different treatment approaches. Ann Surg Oncol 15(6):1585–1593

14. Tseng WH, Martinez SR, Tamurian RM et al (2011) Contiguous organ resection is safe in patients with retroperitoneal sarcoma: an ACS-NSQIP analysis. J Surg Oncol 103(5): 390–394

15. Strauss DC, Hayes AJ, Thway K et al (2010) Surgical management of primary retroperitoneal sarcoma. Br J Surg 97(5):698–706

16. Berselli M, Coppola S, Colombo C et al (2011) Morbidity of left pancreatectomy when associated with multivisceral resection for abdominal mesenchymal neoplasms. JOP 12(2):138–144

17. Nussbaum DP, Speicher PJ, Gulack BC et al (2014) The effect of neoadjuvant radiation therapy on perioperative outcomes among patients undergoing resection of retroperitoneal sarcomas. Surg Oncol 23(3):155–160

18. Bartlett EK, Roses RE, Meise C et al (2014) Preoperative radiation for retroperitoneal sarcoma is not associated with increased early postoperative morbidity. J Surg Oncol 109(6):606–611

19. Kelly KJ, Yoon SS, Kuk D et al (2015) Comparison of perioperative radiation therapy and surgery versus surgery alone in 204 patients with primary retroperitoneal sarcoma: a retrospective 2-institution study. Ann Surg 262(1):156–162

20. Pasquali S, Vohra R, Tsimopoulou I et al (2015) Outcomes following extended surgery for retroperitoneal sarcomas: results from a UK referral centre. Ann Surg Oncol 22(11): 3550–3556

21. Bassi C, Dervenis C, Butturini G et al; International Study Group on Pancreatic Fistula Definition (2005) Postoperative pancreatic fistula: an international study group (ISGPF) definition. Surgery 138(1):8–13

22. Lillemoe KD, Kaushal S, Cameron JL et al (1999) Distal pancreatectomy: indications and outcomes in 235 patients. Ann Surg 229(5):693–698

23. Kleeff J, Diener MK, Z'graggen K et al (2007) Distal pancreatectomy risk factors for surgical failure in 302 consecutive cases. Ann Surg 245(4):573–582

24. Ferrone CR, Warshaw AL, Rattner DW et al (2008) Pancreatic fistula rates after 462 distal pancreatectomies: staplers do not decrease fistula rates. J Gastrointest Surg 12(10): 1691–1697
25. Goh BK, Tan YM, Chung YF et al (2008) Critical appraisal of 232 consecutive distal pancreatectomies with emphasis on risk factors, outcome, and management of the postoperative pancreatic fistula. A 21-year experience at a single institution. Arch Surg 143(10):956–965
26. Knaebel HP, Diener MK, Wente MN et al (2005) Systematic review and meta-analysis of technique for closure of the pancreatic remnant after distal pancreatectomy. Br J Surg 92(5):539–546
27. Irani JL, Ashley SW, Brooks DC et al (2008) Distal pancreatectomy is not associated with increased perioperative morbidity when performed as part of a multivisceral resection. J Gastrointest Surg 12(12):2177–2182
28. Wente MN, Bassi C, Dervenis C et al (2007) Delayed gastric emptying (DGE) after pancreatic surgery: a suggested definition by the International Study Group of Pancreatic Surgery (ISGPS). Surgery 142(5):761–768
29. Fiore M, Colombo C, Locati P et al (2012) Surgical technique, morbidity, and outcome of primary retroperitoneal sarcoma involving inferior vena cava. Ann Surg Oncol 19(2):511–518
30. Radaelli S, Fiore M, Colombo C et al (2016) Vascular resection en-bloc with tumor removal and graft reconstruction is safe and effective in soft tissue sarcoma (STS) of the extremities and retroperitoneum. Surg Oncol 25(3):125–131
31. Hollenbeck ST, Grobmyer SR, Kent KC; Brennan MF (2003) Surgical treatment and outcomes of patients with primary inferior vena cava leiomyosarcoma. J Am Coll Surg 197(4):575–579
32. Ha CP, Rectenwald JE (2018) Inferior vena cava filters: current indications, techniques, and recommendations. Surg Clin North Am 98(2):293–319
33. Tseng WW, Tsao-Wei DD, Callegaro D et al; A Collaborative Effort from the Trans-Atlantic Retroperitoneal Sarcoma Working Group (TARPSWG) (2018) Pancreaticoduodenectomy in the surgical management of primary retroperitoneal sarcoma. Eur J Surg Oncol 44(6):810–815
34. STRASS (EORTC-62092-22092) A phase III randomized study of preoperative radiotherapy plus surgery versus surgery alone for patients with retroperitoneal sarcoma (RPS). ClinicalTrials.gov Identifier: NCT01344018. https://clinicaltrials.gov/ct2/show/ NCT01344018
35. Bonvalot, S, Haas R, Litière C et al (2016) Second safety analysis of a phase III randomized study of preoperative radiotherapy (RT) plus surgery versus surgery alone for patients with retroperitoneal sarcoma (RPS) – EORTC 62092-22092-STRASS. Proceedings of the Connective Tissue Oncology Society. Lisbon, Portugal. 2016 Nov 9–12
36. Sindelar WF, Kinsella TJ, Chen PW et al (1993) Intraoperative radiotherapy in retroperitoneal sarcomas. Final results of a prospective, randomized, clinical trial Arch Surg 128(4):402–410
37. Dziewirski W, Rutkowski P, Nowecki ZI et al (2006) Surgery combined with intraoperative brachytherapy in the treatment of retroperitoneal sarcomas. Ann Surg Oncol 13(2): 245–252
38. Abdelfatah E, Page A, Sacks J et al (2017) Postoperative complications following intraoperative radiotherapy in abdominopelvic malignancy: a single institution analysis of 113 consecutive patients. J Surg Oncol 115(7):883–890
39. Roeder F, Ulrich A, Habl G et al (2014) Clinical phase I/II trial to investigate preoperative dose-escalated intensity-modulated radiation therapy (IMRT) and intraoperative radiation therapy (IORT) in patients with retroperitoneal soft tissue sarcoma: interim analysis. BMC Cancer 14:617

40. Smith MJF, Ridgway PF, Catton CN et al (2014) Combined management of retroperitoneal sarcoma with dose intensification radiotherapy and resection: long-term results of a prospective trial. Radiother Oncol 110(1):165–171
41. Trans-Atlantic RPS Working Group (2015) Management of primary retroperitoneal sarcoma (RPS) in the adult: a consensus approach from the Trans-Atlantic RPS Working Group. Ann Surg Oncol 22(1):256–263
42. Gronchi A, Strauss DC, Miceli R et al (2016) Variability in patterns of recurrence after resection of primary retroperitoneal sarcoma (RPS): a report on 1007 patients from the multi-institutional collaborative RPS working group. Ann Surg 263(5):1002–1009
43. Callegaro D, Miceli R, Brunelli C et al (2015) Long-term morbidity after multivisceral resection for retroperitoneal sarcoma. Br J Surg 102(9):1079–1087
44. Kim DB, Gray R, Li Z et al (2018) Effect of nephrectomy for retroperitoneal sarcoma on post-operative renal function. J Surg Oncol 117(3):425–429
45. Fairweather M, Wang J, Jo VY et al (2017) Incidence and adverse prognostic implications of histopathologic organ invasion in primary retroperitoneal sarcoma. J Am Coll Surg 224(5):876–883
46. Russo P, Kim Y, Ravindran S et al (1997) Nephrectomy during operative management of retroperitoneal sarcoma. Ann Surg Oncol 4(5):421–424
47. Mussi C, Colombo P, Bertuzzi A et al (2011) Retroperitoneal sarcoma: is it time to change the surgical policy? Ann Surg Oncol 18(8):2136–2142
48. Hull MA, Niemierko A, Haynes AB et al (2015) Post-operative renal function following nephrectomy as part of en bloc resection of retroperitoneal sarcoma (RPS). J Surg Oncol 112(1):98–102
49. Wong P, Kassam Z, Springer AN et al (2017) Long-term quality of life of retroperitoneal sarcoma patients treated with pre-operative radiotherapy and surgery. Cureus 9(10):e1764
50. Fiore M, Callegaro D, Lenna S et al (2017) Quality of life (QoL) and pain in primary retroperitoneal sarcoma (RPS): preliminary data from a prospective observational study. Ann Surg Oncol 24(Suppl 1):S165

Major Vascular Resection in Retroperitoneal Surgery

7

Ferdinando C.M. Cananzi, Laura Ruspi, Jacopo Galvanin, and Vittorio Quagliuolo

7.1   Introduction

Infiltration of major blood vessels has long been a criterion of non-resectability in cancer surgery. In recent decades, the improvements in surgical technique and perioperative management, along with a better understanding of the biology and natural history of the disease, have led to reconsider this principle in several types of tumors. Indeed, the so-called *oncovascular surgery* (i.e., surgery where cancer resection needs concomitant ligation or reconstruction of a major vessel) has been employed with favorable outcome – when planned within a multidisciplinary therapeutic approach – in urological cancer, pancreatic carcinoma, limb and retroperitoneal sarcoma (RPS) [1]. As reported elsewhere in this monograph, complete surgical resection is the cornerstone of the treatment of RPS, frequently requiring complex multivisceral resection. An attempt to categorize the rationale for structure resection has been recently proposed by Fairweather et al. using a six-tier system including: 1) suspected organ invasion/tumor origin; 2) tumor involving end-organ vascular supply; 3) tumor encasement of organ (organ involvement larger than 180°); 4) tumor adherent to organ; 5) tumor adjacent to organ/required for microscopic complete resection (R0/R1 resection); 6) other cause (i.e., iatrogenic injury requiring resection, incidental resection for another reason) [2]. This classification may also apply to major vessels which are usually resected because RPS may either originate from them or secondarily invade or encase them (category 1, 3 and 4). Besides rationale, major vascular resections are not rare, having been performed in 143

F.C.M. Cananzi (✉)
Surgical Oncology Unit, Department of Surgery, Humanitas Clinical and Research Center
Rozzano, Milan, Italy
e-mail: ferdinando.cananzi@humanitas.it

V. Quagliuolo, A. Gronchi (Eds), *Current Treatment of Retroperitoneal Sarcomas*, Updates in Surgery
DOI: 10.1007/978-88-470-3980-3_7, © Springer-Verlag Italia 2019

(14%) out of 1007 patients with primary RPS analyzed in the recently published study from the Trans-Atlantic Retroperitoneal Sarcoma Working Group [3].

7.2   Preoperative Assessment

The radiological staging of RPS involving major blood vessels does not differ from the method employed in other RPS, with computed tomography and magnetic resonance imaging needed to identify possible distant metastases and to evaluate local tumor extension. When the inferior vena cava (IVC) is involved, close attention should also be paid in defining the degree of lumen obstruction and the presence of collateral veins, which are conditions that may significantly affect the surgical strategy.

Before establishing the proper management of RPS requiring oncovascular resection, the estimated prognosis should be accurately balanced with expected morbidity. On one hand, stage (primary or metastatic or recurrent), histology and supposed origin of the sarcoma (i.e., tumor arising from the vessels or retroperitoneal soft tissue tumor invading/encasing the vessels) are the most important factors affecting prognosis and possible oncological benefit. On the other hand, the expected morbidity is mainly due to the extent and type of vascular resection and concomitant cumulative organ removal. Moreover, the patient's performance status, comorbidities and possible functional impairment must also be taken into consideration and must be counterbalanced with the risk of an incomplete resection in order to plan the most appropriate treatment [4–6].

7.3   Primary Vascular Sarcomas

Basically, primary retroperitoneal vascular sarcomas are visceral sarcomas originating from the wall of the vessel (artery or vein). Primary sarcomas of the IVC are mostly represented by leiomyosarcoma (LMS), which is a rare neoplasia of the smooth muscle of the vein wall, accounting for approximately 0.5% of soft tissue sarcomas, with fewer than 390 cases reported in the literature. It occurs more commonly in females and the median age at presentation is about 55 years [7–9].

These tumors could be classified according to their location as proposed by Hollenbeck: upper (tumors arising in the segment of the IVC from the right atrium to the hepatic veins), middle (from the hepatic to the renal veins), or lower (below the renal veins) IVC sarcomas. [10].

Clinical presentation may vary significantly and it is usually conditioned by the tumor location: lower sarcoma can cause lower extremity edema and abdominal pain; LMS of the middle part may provoke abdominal pain and sometimes causes reno-vascular hypertension; tumor arising in the proximal segment can originate a Budd-Chiari syndrome with symptoms including abdominal distention, nausea, vomiting, hepatomegaly, ascites, and jaundice, in consideration of the hepatic vein involvement [11].

Primary LMS usually grows via intra-luminal or extra-luminal pattern and local spread. In most cases, imaging studies show an IVC filled with tumor, as well as extraluminal growth in the retroperitoneum. When a pronounced extraluminal extension is detected, the differential diagnosis between LMS of the IVC and LMS of retroperitoneal soft tissue involving the IVC may be particularly challenging.

Complete surgical resection is the cornerstone of the treatment of primary LMS of IVC, but the majority of patients will finally fail mainly due to distant recurrence with 5-year disease-free survival rates ranging from 7% to 44%. However, the overall survival (OS) was generally higher with 5-year survival rates of 33–67% [8, 10–14]. Advanced age, large tumor size, resection of adjacent organs and surgical margin status were described as independent prognostic factors [15]. In the metastatic setting, although there are few published data, surgical resection of recurrent/metastatic disease – when feasible – seems to prolong OS [8, 9].

Primary malignant sarcomas of the aorta are extremely rare, as less than 200 cases have been described in the literature, with undifferentiated tumor histology, leiomyosarcoma, fibrosarcoma, hemangioendothelioma, myxoid sarcomas and angiosarcoma representing the more common subtypes. The thoracic aorta is slightly more frequently affected than the abdominal aorta; the aortic arch was involved only in few cases. Patients frequently present with symptoms and signs related to thromboembolic events to abdominal viscera, brain and extremities (mesenteric infarction, acute arterial embolization, claudication, abdominal pain, back pain). In some cases, primary sarcoma of the aorta may mimic a diffuse thrombotic disease [16–18].

The prognosis of this aggressive sarcoma is dismal with an estimated 1-year, 3-year, and 5-year OS of 46.7%, 17.1%, and 8.8%, respectively [19]. Mortality is mainly due to the above-mentioned tumor-related complications and distant spreading of disease, which occurs in about 80% of patients and involves bone, lung, liver, kidney, and skin [17, 19, 20].

7.4 Retroperitoneal Soft Tissue Sarcomas Involving Major Vessels

Compared with primary vascular sarcoma, a retroperitoneal soft tissue sarcoma secondarily infiltrating or encasing vessels is a more frequent condition requiring major vascular resection. As expected, LMS and liposarcoma are the most frequent histotypes accounting for vascular involvement but other subtypes such as undifferentiated pleomorphic sarcoma, clear cell sarcoma and synovial sarcoma have also been reported in the literature [5, 21]. The main clinical features of the different kinds of RPS are examined in depth elsewhere in this monograph.

The high heterogeneity of RPS and the pronounced difference in data reporting make it difficult to assess whether vascular invasion should be considered as a sign of enhanced malignancy or as a "simple" reflection of the anatomic location and large size of RPS. However, several studies have demonstrated that major vessel involvement is not a contraindication for resecting a RPS with curative intent [4, 5, 21, 22]. The outcomes reported in some of the most representative surgical series are shown in Table 7.1.

These results reported after oncovascular surgery for RPS trace what has been observed in other solid tumors such as pancreatic and rectal carcinoma, in which long-term survival seems not to be affected by the need for resection of the portal vein and aortoiliac axis, respectively [23–26].

In the study by Bertrand et al., reporting on about 22 patients who underwent vascular resection for RPS, there was no statistically significant difference in terms of progression-free survival and local recurrence between patients with histologically proven vessel invasion and those with simple encasement [5]. Accordingly, in the matched case-control study from Stanford University including 50 patients (27 RPS) undergoing sarcoma resection with vascular reconstruction and 100 patients (54 RPS) without vascular reconstruction, 5-year OS and 5-year local recurrence rates were similar in the two groups (59% vs. 53% and 51% vs. 54%, respectively). Also, OS was significantly affected by high tumor grading and presence of synchronous metastases but it was not hampered by the presence of histology-proven vessel wall invasion. Similarly, completeness of resection and grading were found to be major prognostic factors in most of the other relevant studies published so far [4, 5, 21, 22].

Taken together, these data lead to consider vascular involvement as a relevant surgical issue to be managed in order to achieve improved local control rather than a negative prognostic factor per se. Nevertheless, the high incidence of distant metastases reported in patients who underwent vessel resection for a soft tissue sarcoma suggests that vascular invasion should be at least considered as an indirect marker of biological aggressiveness requiring multidisciplinary evaluation and effective systemic therapy when appropriate [6, 27]. Indeed, the majority of patients analyzed in the aforementioned studies harbored a high-grade RPS.

Major vascular structures require resection when sarcoma originates from them or invades or encases them. As mentioned, in this scenario the choice of performing such a complex resection mainly depends on the balance between estimated prognosis and expected surgical morbidity and mortality.

Table 7.1 Surgical data and results of the main studies on surgery for RPS involving major blood vessels

Study	N of patients	Follow-up (years)	Years	Type of resection	Reconstruction rate	Type of reconstruction	Patency rate	5-years LRFS	5-years DMFS	5-years OS
Dzsinich et al. 1992 [49]	13	ns	1957–1990	A=1 V=13	A=100% V=54%	V: PTFE/Dacron/Vein/Primary: 28%; 14%; 14%; 43%	ns	15%	38%	38%*
Ridwelski et al. 2001 [50]	5	ns	1993–1999	IVC=5	V: 80%	PTFE/NS: 75%; 25%	ns	0%	40%	60%*
Hollenbeck et al. 2003 [10]	21	2	1982–2002	IVC=21	V=52%	Primary/PTFE/Vein: 70%; 20%; 10%	80%#	ns	ns	33%
Schwarzbach et al. 2006 [21]	25	1.6	1988–2004	A=9 V=20	A=100% V=75%	A: PTFE/Dacron/Primary: 22%; 67%; 11% V: PTFE/Dacron/Primary/Vein: 63%; 12%; 19%; 6%	A=89% V=94%#	ns	ns	56%
Kieffer et al. 2006 [11]	19	3.6	1979–2004	IVC=19	V=75%	PTFE/Primary: 93%; 7%	90%#	DFS: 33%		35%
Ito et al. 2007 [8]	20	3.4	1990–2006	IVC=20	V=85%	Primary/Synthetic graft: 71%; 29%	ns	66%	41%	62%
Fiore et al. 2012 [14]	15	2.6	2004–2011	IVC=15	V=73%	Homograft/PTFE: 73%; 27%	60%#	80%	74%	80%
Poultsides et al. 2015 [22]	27	2	2000–2014	A=12 V=20	A=100% V=62%	A: PTFE/Synthetic graft/Dacron: 25%; 33%; 42% V: Vein/PTFE/Synthetic graft/Primary: 10%; 45%; 20%; 25%	86% (5 years)	80%	38%	59%
Radaelli et al. 2016 [27]	42	2.7	2000–2013	A=12 V=30	A=100% V=64%	A: PTFE: 100% V: PTFE/Cadaveric graft: 48%; 52%	A=92% V=82%#	88%	42%	62%
Bertrand et al. 2016 [5]	31	ns	2000–2013	A=14 V=31	A/V=93%	Prosthetic graft/Primary/Reimplantation: 76%; 7%; 17%	A/V=100%#	29%	84%	61% (3 years)
Cananzi et al. 2016 [9]	11	7.7	2000–2012	IVC=11	V=73%	Primary/Synthetic graft: 50%; 50%	ns	ns	10%	60%
Wortmann et al. 2017 [4]	20	ns	1994–2014	A=20 V=13	A=100% V=15%	A: Autologous/Synthetic graft: 30%; 70% V: PTFE: 100%	A=88% V=0% (2 years)	10%	15%	69% (2 years)

LRFS, local recurrence-free survival; *DMFS*, distant metastasis-free survival; *DFS*, disease-free survival; *OS*, overall survival; *ns*, not specified; *IVC*, inferior vena cava; *A*, artery; *V*, vein; *PTFE*, polytetrafluoroethylene; * total percentage of survivors; # overall patency.

However, in several cases the sarcoma is only adherent to the vessel, which is pushed by the tumor but not actually infiltrated. In these patients an oncovascular resection may represent an overtreatment that adds morbidity with no real benefit. In Fairweather et al.'s recent study, including 118 patients operated on for primary RPS, 17 patients (14%) needed a vascular resection of major retroperitoneal vessels (aorta, IVC, renal or iliac) mainly due to suspected invasion/tumor origin followed by tumor adherent to organ and encasement of the organ. At the pathology review, 70% of the removed vessels demonstrated evidence of histopathologic organ invasion (HOI). Importantly, when all the resected organs were considered, the HOI rate observed in the study dropped to 25%, proving that a more restrictive resection policy was employed in dealing with major blood vessels [2].

Schwarzbach et al. reported on about 25 patients with RPS including eight patients with primary and 17 with secondary major vascular involvement. Of the latter, 11 (65%) had vessel wall infiltration at pathologic examination [21]. These data are similar to those shown in the matched case-control study by Poultsides et al. where a histologic vessel invasion was registered in 21 (62%) of 34 patients and was more common in resected veins (18/26, 69%) than arteries (3/16, 19%) [22]. These high rates of HOI should not lead to overestimate the actual need for vessel resection in RPS, considering that both primary vascular sarcoma and RPS secondarily involving vessels were analyzed and that no data about operations where the vessels were just dissected (i.e., not resected) were provided in these studies.

Indeed, vascular adventitia may represent an anatomical barrier when left on the side of the tumor and a safe plane for vessel dissection limiting perioperative morbidity without increasing the risk of local recurrence [28, 29]. Also, there is no evidence suggesting that a systematic vascular resection may be beneficial in terms of local control of the disease and OS [6]. On the contrary, major vascular resection is a well-known procedure associated with increased morbidity almost doubling the risk of postoperative adverse events [22, 30].

Basically, dissection of the tumor under the adventitia should be attempted when approaching all major retroperitoneal vessels, unless widely encased and/ or overtly infiltrated. However, it is worth noting that sometimes peritumoral inflammation and desmoplastic reaction are hard to differentiate from true vascular wall invasion [21, 31–34]. Moreover, a blood vessel resection may be required to prevent or control accidental vascular injury during the dissection of a pushing tumor from a weakened vascular wall.

7.5   Recurrent/Metastatic Retroperitoneal Sarcomas

The management of metastatic/recurrent RPS is discussed elsewhere in this monograph but it should basically follow the recommendations of the Trans-

Atlantic Retroperitoneal Sarcoma Working Group (TARPSWG) [35]. Herein, it is important to highlight the role of tumor biology, the overall burden of disease and the patient's performance status as main determinants in the decision-making process. Generally, the resection of a local recurrence involving major vessels should be restricted to carefully selected patients and performed within a multidisciplinary approach with a curative intent in specialized centers, as the expected survival benefits are usually modest [35, 36]. Moreover, the need for resecting an involved intestinal tract – which frequently occurs in RPS recurrence – may represent an additional concern when a concomitant oncovascular resection could be required [6].

7.6   Surgical Technique in Major Vascular Resection

Once the decision of a vascular resection has been made, it is fundamental to plan the surgical strategy and the possible type of reconstruction, which should be tailored according to extent of resection and to the type of resected vessel (artery versus vein). A possible treatment algorithm is showed in Fig. 7.1.

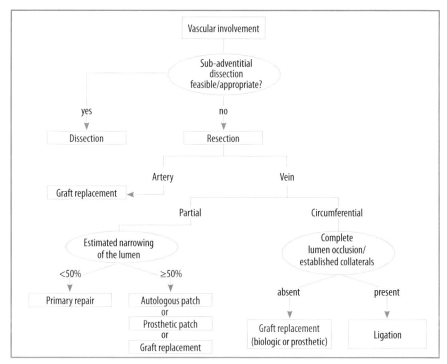

Fig. 7.1 Proposed algorithm of surgical treatment in patients affected by retroperitoneal sarcoma with major vessel involvement

7.6.1 Arterial Reconstructions

As previously reported, primary sarcomas of the aorta are exceptional. More often, this vessel is secondarily involved or encased by other malignancies; in these cases, also the IVC is frequently affected [6]. When arterial resection is required, a primary anastomosis is rarely feasible because of the extent of the resection performed to obtain free margins. Therefore, orthotopic synthetic prostheses are usually preferred to restore continuity (Table 7.1, Fig. 7.2). Radaelli et al. employed a prosthetic polytetrafluoroethylene (PTFE) graft with or without integrated rings for reconstruction of large caliber arteries, with a patency rate higher than 90% [27]. Prosthetic reconstruction with a Dacron graft has also been described in a series of seven patients who underwent resection for primary angiosarcoma of the aorta; unfortunately, very limited data on patency and effectiveness of this reconstruction are available given the extremely high

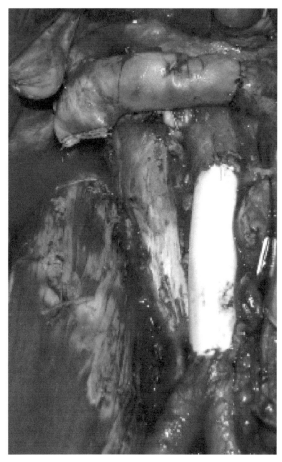

Fig. 7.2 Prosthetic replacement of the aorta with concomitant ligation of the inferior vena cava and reconstruction of the venous reno-caval confluence using a banked venous homograft

mortality reported in this series, with a median survival around 14 months [16]. Schwarzbach et al. reported on the use of synthetic prostheses (expanded PTFE or Dacron) preferably in anatomic position for aortic resection, while reversed great saphenous vein was considered in the reconstruction of visceral or iliac vessels [21] (Table 7.1).

In a series of 20 patients with RPS, Wortmann et al. reported on six patients requiring aortic resection; in one patient the infrarenal aorta was ligated and arterial flow to the limbs was then guaranteed by fashioning of an extra-anatomic axillary-bifemoral bypass [4].

In patients requiring iliac artery resection and concomitant colic resection, a cross-femoral arterial bypass may be preferred in order to avoid proximity of vascular and intestinal anastomoses [6]. The use of silver-containing prostheses or grafts treated with antibiotic has also been described by Schwarzbach et al. when a large bowel resection was planned; in their series only one graft infection occurred (due to a perforated sigmoid diverticulitis) and the overall patency rate in arterial reconstruction was 89% (median follow-up 19.3 months) [21].

The encasement of the superior mesenteric vessels is generally considered a potential criterion of non-resectability in RPS surgery. However, in tumors extending into the mesenteric root a segmental resection of the superior mesenteric artery may be exceptionally performed [6]: in such cases, a primary anastomosis, reinsertion of the artery or a small diameter graft (autologous or synthetic) may be used for vascular reconstruction [21]. Such an aggressive approach may be justified only in primary tumors with a proximal encasement of the superior mesenteric artery [6].

7.6.2   Venous Reconstructions

The first reported resection of an IVC leiomyosarcoma on veno-venous bypass was performed in 1993 [37] but surgical reconstruction of the IVC has not yet been standardized [6, 38]. The surgical strategy in reconstructing the IVC should take into account the site of the tumor, the extent of resection (partial or circumferential), the patency of the vein and the presence of well-established venous collaterals. The options for management include primary or patch repair, ligation, or replacement with interposition of a graft (synthetic or biologic).

Primary repair is routinely used in partial resection of the IVC wall and it can be performed when <50% narrowing of the lumen is expected [38]. Instead, a prosthetic or biologic patch (autologous venous graft, fascio-peritoneal patch) can be employed in wider partial wall resection of the IVC [21, 39]. Primary repair or autologous patching should be preferred – whenever it is possible – as they do not require lifelong anticoagulation and they are less prone to lower limb edema and risk of infection, which is a major issue especially when intestinal resections are also required [40].

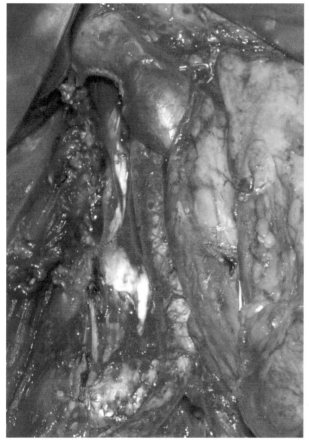

Fig. 7.3 Inferior vena cava resection without reconstruction (i.e., ligation) preserving the left renal vein confluence (note the enlarged gonadal vein)

IVC ligation is usually feasible and well tolerated when the vessel lumen is already occluded; in such cases it is mandatory to preserve the collateral venous drainage during surgical maneuvers [41]. On one hand, this approach prevents the occurrence of pulmonary thromboembolism and does not require lifelong anticoagulation, as well as avoiding graft-related complications [6]. On the other hand, significant edema of lower extremities has been reported in up to 50% of patients undergoing IVC ligation [42]. Our surgical policy usually favors vein ligation without reconstruction when the preoperative study demonstrated a non-patent IVC, confirmed by the intraoperative finding [9] (Figs. 7.2, 7.3). However, there is still no agreement on this issue, since different surgical policies and incidence rates of lower limb edema are described in the literature [9, 10].

When ligation is not indicated and the IVC needs to be replaced, several reconstruction techniques can be employed. The positioning of a PTFE prosthetic graft is one of the most common methods for replacing the IVC [14, 38, 43] (Fig. 7.4).

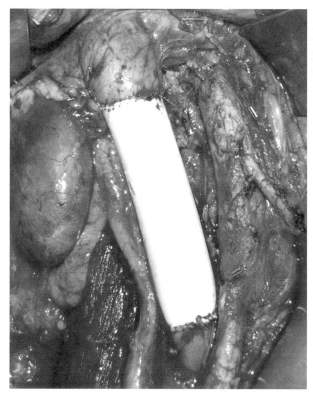

Fig. 7.4 Inferior vena cava reconstruction with prosthetic polytetrafluoroethylene graft

To prevent the occlusion of the graft – which is one of the main concerns in venous reconstruction – some authors suggested ring-reinforced PTFE grafts while others reported the fashioning of an inguinal arteriovenous fistula in order to enhance blood flow and pressure within the graft [44]. Another rare but potentially life-threatening complication following prosthetic reconstruction is graft infection, whose incidence is higher when concomitant bowel resection is performed [14, 43]. In this scenario, omental interposition between the graft and resected viscera may be helpful in lowering the infection rate [44].

Fiore et al. were the first to report IVC replacement with a banked venous homograft after resection of a primary LMS [39] (Fig. 7.5a,b). IVC replacement with homograft presents many advantages in comparison to prosthetic grafts, being associated with a lower risk of infection and not requiring life-long anticoagulation. Moreover, it showed a relatively mild rate of occlusion (2–9% vs. 16–40% of PTFE grafts) which could be probably due to less pronounced immune response against the venous homograft [39, 45–47]. This approach seems to be the best way to IVC reconstruction but its wide diffusion is hindered by limited availability since harvesting from multi-organ donors is not a routine procedure [39].

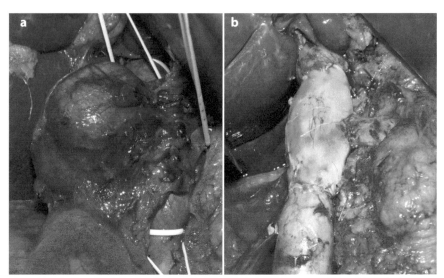

Fig. 7.5 Inferior vena cava resection (**a**) with concomitant reconstruction (**b**) with banked venous homograft and re-implantation of the left renal vein

Whenever IVC resection is required, particular attention to renal vessels and their management needs to be paid. If the right kidney is preserved, the right renal vein has to be re-implanted since collateral venous outflow is generally lacking on this side [38]. Conversely, the sectioning of the left renal vein may be tolerated as collaterals are normally represented by adrenal, lumbar, gonadal and diaphragmatic veins [6].

In cases of sarcoma involving the iliac vessels, a complete resection may include a portion of peritoneum on one side and of the psoas muscle on the other [28]. The iliac arterial axis is usually restored by means of prosthetic grafts, while the need to replace the vein is controversial. Iliac vein ligation without reconstruction is often well tolerated because of the existence of frequent collaterals. Vein reconstruction may be recommended when a concomitant resection of the great saphenous vein, the femoral vein and the venous collaterals in the adductor muscles is performed, in order to avoid serious subsequent venous disease [4, 48]. Techniques described for IVC reconstruction can apply to iliac vein replacement as well.

7.7   Morbidity and Mortality

It is well acknowledged from retrospective studies that major vascular resections for RPS significantly increase postoperative morbidity. In the large report from the TARPSWG, major vascular resections were associated with a two-fold increase in the risk of severe adverse events; this odds ratio was higher than that for pancreaticoduodenectomy and simultaneous resection of the colon, kidney, spleen and pancreas [30].

In a review of patients who underwent surgery for IVC LMS, Wachtel et al. reported a 30-day operative mortality of 1.9%, an overall complication rate of 24.7% (the most common complications being lower extremity edema and renal failure), and a re-operation rate of 3.1% [12]. The morbidity rate in major vascular resection is often higher than 30%. Quinones-Baldrich et al. reported major complications in 10.6% of patients, with no difference among the types of IVC reconstruction [38]. Bertrand et al. reported major complications in 19.3%, with a need for reoperation in 16%; however, no mortality was observed in his series [5]. Many authors reported a patency rate higher than 80% after 2 years from surgery (Table 7.1); rates are higher for arterial reconstruction with Radaelli et al. observing no occlusion in 89% of cases and Schwarzbach et al. describing a patency rate of about 89% [4, 21, 27] (Table 7.1).

As regards long term outcomes, survival rates of the main studies are shown in Table 7.1. However, data are limited and not easily comparable due to the rarity of the disease and the heterogeneity in the surgical management.

7.8 Conclusions

Although representing a technical challenge, major blood vessel involvement is not a contraindication for surgical resection with curative intent of RPS. Subadventitial dissection should be regarded as the first approach; however, oncovascular resection could be appropriate in primary sarcomas of the vessels and in RPS with wide secondary involvement of vascular structures in order to improve the completeness of resection. The proper surgical strategy, including extent of resection and type of reconstruction, should be tailored to each patient according to tumor biology and balancing estimated survival benefits with expected morbidity. Therefore, it is strongly recommended that major vascular resections for RPS should be performed in a specialized sarcoma center after having been carefully discussed by a multidisciplinary tumor board.

References

1. Ghosh J, Bhowmick A, Baguneid M (2011) Oncovascular surgery. Eur J Surg Oncol 37(12):1017–1024
2. Fairweather M, Wang J, Jo VY et al (2018) Surgical management of primary retroperitoneal sarcomas: rationale for selective organ resection. Ann Surg Oncol 25(1):98–106

3. Gronchi A, Strauss DC, Miceli R et al (2016) Variability in patterns of recurrence after resection of primary retroperitoneal sarcoma (RPS): a report on 1007 patients from the multi-institutional collaborative RPS working group. Ann Surg 263(5):1002–1009

4. Wortmann M, Alldinger I, Böckler D et al (2017) Vascular reconstruction after retroperitoneal and lower extremity sarcoma resection. Eur J Surg Oncol 43(2):407–415

5. Bertrand MM, Carrère S, Delmond L et al (2016) Oncovascular compartmental resection for retroperitoneal soft tissue sarcoma with vascular involvement. J Vasc Surg 64(4):1033–1041

6. Tzanis D, Bouhadiba T, Gaignard E, Bonvalot S (2018) Major vascular resections in retroperitoneal sarcoma. J Surg Oncol 117(1):42–47

7. Perl L, Virchow R (1871) Ein Fall von Sarkom der Vena cava inferior. Arch f path Anat 53(4):378–383

8. Ito H, Hornick JL, Bertagnolli MM et al (2007) Leiomyosarcoma of the inferior vena cava: survival after aggressive management. Ann Surg Oncol 14(12):3534–3541

9. Cananzi FC, Mussi C, Bordoni MG et al (2016) Role of surgery in the multimodal treatment of primary and recurrent leiomyosarcoma of the inferior vena cava. J Surg Oncol 114(1):44–49

10. Hollenbeck ST, Grobmyer SR, Kent KC, Brennan MF (2003) Surgical treatment and outcomes of patients with primary inferior vena cava leiomyosarcoma. J Am Coll Surg 197(4):575–579

11. Kieffer E, Alaoui M, Piette JC et al (2006) Leiomyosarcoma of the inferior vena cava: experience in 22 cases. Ann Surg 244(2): 289–295

12. Wachtel H, Jackson BM, Bartlett EK et al (2015) Resection of primary leiomyosarcoma of the inferior vena cava (IVC) with reconstruction: a case series and review of the literature. J Surg Oncol 111(3):328–333

13. Mingoli A, Cavallaro A, Sapienza P et al (1996) International registry of inferior vena cava leiomyosarcoma: analysis of a world series on 218 patients. Anticancer Res 16(5B):3201–3205

14. Fiore M, Colombo C, Locati P et al (2012) Surgical technique, morbidity, and outcome of primary retroperitoneal sarcoma involving inferior vena cava. Ann Surg Oncol 19(2):511–518

15. Wachtel H, Gupta M, Bartlett EK et al (2015) Outcomes after resection of leiomyosarcomas of the inferior vena cava: a pooled data analysis of 377 cases. Surg Oncol 24(1):21–27

16. Fatima J, Duncan AA, Maleszewski JJ et al (2013) Primary angiosarcoma of the aorta, great vessels, and the heart. J Vasc Surg 57(3):756–764

17. Seelig MH, Klingler PJ, Oldenburg A, Blackshear JL (1998) Angiosarcoma of the aorta: report of a case and review of the literature. J Vasc Surg 28(4):732–737

18. Böhner H, Luther B, Braunstein S et al (2003) Primary malignant tumors of the aorta: clinical presentation, treatment, and course of different entities. J Vasc Surg 38(6): 1430–1433

19. Rusthoven CG, Liu AK, Bui MM et al (2014) Sarcomas of the aorta: a systematic review and pooled analysis of published reports. Ann Vasc Surg 28(2):515–525

20. Chiche L, Mongrédien B, Brocheriou I, Kieffer E (2003) Primary tumors of the thoracoabdominal aorta: surgical treatment of 5 patients and review of the literature. Ann Vasc Surg 17(4):354–364

21. Schwarzbach MH, Hormann Y, Hinz U et al (2006) Clinical results of surgery for retroperitoneal sarcoma with major blood vessel involvement. J Vasc Surg 44(1):46–55

22. Poultsides GA, Tran TB, Zambrano E et al (2015) Sarcoma resection with and without vascular reconstruction: a matched case-control study. Ann Surg 262(4):632–640

23. Harrison LE, Klimstra DS, Brennan MF (1996) Isolated portal vein involvement in pancreatic adenocarcinoma. A contraindication for resection? Ann Surg 224(3):342–347

24. Kelly KJ, Winslow E, Kooby D et al (2013) Vein involvement during pancreaticoduodenectomy: is there a need for redefinition of "borderline resectable disease"? J Gastrointest Surg 17(7):1209–1217

25. Norton JA, Harris EJ, Chen Y et al (2011) Pancreatic endocrine tumors with major vascular abutment, involvement, or encasement and indication for resection. Arch Surg 146(6):724–732

26. Abdelsattar ZM, Mathis KL, Colibaseanu DT et al (2013) Surgery for locally advanced recurrent colorectal cancer involving the aortoiliac axis: can we achieve R0 resection and long-term survival? Dis Colon Rectum 56(6):711–716

27. Radaelli S, Fiore M, Colombo C et al (2016) Vascular resection en-bloc with tumor removal and graft reconstruction is safe and effective in soft tissue sarcoma (STS) of the extremities and retroperitoneum. Surg Oncol 25(3):125–131

28. Bonvalot S, Raut CP, Pollock RE et al (2012) Technical considerations in surgery for retroperitoneal sarcomas: position paper from E-Surge, a master class in sarcoma surgery, and EORTC-STBSG. Ann Surg Oncol 19(9):2981–2991

29. Trans-Atlantic RPS Working Group (2015) Management of primary retroperitoneal sarcoma (RPS) in the adult: a consensus approach from the Trans-Atlantic RPS Working Group. Ann Surg Oncol 22(1):256–263

30. MacNeill AJ, Gronchi A, Miceli R et al (2018) Postoperative morbidity after radical resection of primary retroperitoneal sarcoma: a report from the Trans-Atlantic RPS Working Group. Ann Surg 267(5):959–964

31. Schwarzbach MH, Hormann Y, Hinz U et al (2005) Results of limb-sparing surgery with vascular replacement for soft tissue sarcoma in the lower extremity. J Vasc Surg 42(1):88–97

32. Carpenter SG, Stone WM, Bower TC et al (2011) Surgical management of tumors invading the aorta and major arterial structures. Ann Vasc Surg 25(8):1026–1035

33. Tseng JF, Raut CP, Lee JE et al (2004) Pancreaticoduodenectomy with vascular resection: margin status and survival duration. J Gastrointest Surg 8(8):935–949

34. Roder JD, Stein HJ, Siewert JR (1996) Carcinoma of the periampullary region: who benefits from portal vein resection? Am J Surg 171(1):170–174; discussion 174–175

35. Trans-Atlantic RPS Working Group (2016) Management of recurrent retroperitoneal sarcoma (RPS) in the adult: a consensus approach from the Trans-Atlantic RPS Working Group. Ann Surg Oncol 23(11):3531–3540

36. MacNeill AJ, Miceli R, Strauss DC et al (2017) Post-relapse outcomes after primary extended resection of retroperitoneal sarcoma: a report from the Trans-Atlantic RPS Working Group. Cancer 123(11):1971–1978

37. Yanaga K, Okadome K, Ito H et al (1993) Graft replacement of pararenal inferior vena cava for leiomyosarcoma with the use of venous bypass. Surgery 113(1):109–112

38. Quinones-Baldrich W, Alktaifi A, Eilber F, Eilber F (2012) Inferior vena cava resection and reconstruction for retroperitoneal tumor excision. J Vasc Surg 55(5):1386–1393

39. Fiore M, Locati P, Mussi C et al (2008) Banked venous homograft replacement of the inferior vena cava for primary leiomyosarcoma. Eur J Surg Oncol 34(6):720–724

40. Suzman MS, Smith AJ, Brennan MF (2000) Fascio-peritoneal patch repair of the IVC: a workhorse in search of work? J Am Coll Surg 191(2):218–220

41. Dull BZ, Smith B, Tefera G, Weber S (2013) Surgical management of retroperitoneal leiomyosarcoma arising from the inferior vena cava. J Gastrointest Surg 17(12): 2166–2171

42. Daylami R, Amiri A, Goldsmith B et al (2010) Inferior vena cava leiomyosarcoma: is reconstruction necessary after resection? J Am Coll Surg 210(2):185–190

43. Bower TC, Nagorney DM, Cherry KJ Jr et al (2000) Replacement of the inferior vena cava for malignancy: an update. J Vasc Surg 31(2):270–281

44. Hardwigsen J, Baqué P, Crespy B et al (2001) Resection of the inferior vena cava for neoplasms with or without prosthetic replacement: a 14-patient series. Ann Surg 233(2):242–249

45. Lim JH, Sohn SH, Sung YW et al (2014) Banked vena caval homograft replacement of the inferior vena cava for primary leiomyosarcoma. Korean J Thorac Cardiovasc Surg 47(5):473–477

46. Di Benedetto F, D'Amico G, Montalti R et al (2012) Banked depopulated vena caval homograft: a new strategy to restore caval continuity. Surg Innov 19(1):NP5–NP9
47. Faenza A, Ferraro A, Gigli M et al (2005) Vascular homografts for vessel substitution in skeletal and soft tissue sarcomas of the limbs. Transplant Proc 37(6):2692–2693
48. Matsushita M, Kuzuya A, Mano N et al (2001) Sequelae after limb-sparing surgery with major vascular resection for tumor of the lower extremity. J Vasc Surg 33(4):694–699
49. Dzsinich C, Gloviczki P, Van Heerden JA et al (1992) Primary venous leiomyosarcoma: a rare but lethal disease. J Vasc Surg 15(4):592–603
50. Ridwelski K, Rudolph S, Meyer F et al (2001) Primary sarcoma of the inferior vena cava: review of diagnosis, treatment, and outcomes in a case series. Int Surg 86(3):184–190

Pattern and Management of Recurrent Retroperitoneal Liposarcoma

8

Elisabetta Pennacchioli, Massimo Barberis, and Stefania Rizzo

8.1 Introduction

Despite optimal resection of primary retroperitoneal liposarcoma (RLPS), overall local/abdominal recurrence is common. Moreover, local recurrence in RLPS is the most common cause of mortality, with up to 75% of deaths occurring in the absence of distant metastasis [1, 2]. A high proportion of recurrences occur late, even after five years. As in other soft tissue sarcomas, histological subtype and complete resection are the most important prognostic factors for recurrence-free survival (RFS) and overall survival (OS), and influence significantly the outcome of patients who experience recurrence.

Due to the complexity of the surgical approach to retroperitoneal sarcoma (RPS), patients who have had an incomplete resection of their primary tumor or who experience recurrent disease after primary resection are typically then referred to a tertiary care institution with significant experience in the management of sarcoma. Among these centers, however, consensus on the optimal management of these patients is still debated. Decision-making in cases of recurrent or residual RLPS is a challenge for both clinicians and patients and data from the literature do not completely recognize prognostic features to guide patient selection.

It is known that RPS accounts for 15% of all sarcomas, and 50% are RLPS. Based on the evidence that different histologic subtypes have different patterns and timing of recurrence following resection of primary RPS and that the distribution of histological subtypes in recurrent RPS is distinct from that of primary RPS [1–6], we can assume that this is true also per RLPS. Few studies

E. Pennacchioli (✉)
Soft Tissue Sarcoma and Rare Tumors Surgical Division, European Institute of Oncology
Milan, Italy
e-mail: elisabetta.pennacchioli@ieo.it

V. Quagliuolo, A. Gronchi (Eds), *Current Treatment of Retroperitoneal Sarcomas*,
Updates in Surgery
DOI: 10.1007/978-88-470-3980-3_8, © Springer-Verlag Italia 2019

report that a less aggressive surgical approach for low-grade RLPS does not lead to worse OS compared to other series treated with a more extended approach. This is another topic of debate, as recent evidence from large series [7] suggests that an extended approach is more appropriate for low-intermediate grade tumors only. In general, recurrent RPS is associated with a worse prognosis than primary RPS.

8.2   Biology of Recurrence in Retroperitoneal Liposarcoma

The rates and patterns of failure of all RPS histologic subtypes are related, from a clinical point of view, to a small number of factors: patient characteristics, tumor features, and surgical variables. In RLPS the key biologic features of prognosis are histologic subtype, grading and margin status of primary resection [5, 7–9].

8.2.1   Role of Histologic Subtype

According to the WHO Classification of Tumors of Soft Tissue and Bone [10], the histologic tumor subtypes are the following:
- well-differentiated liposarcoma (WDLPS);
- dedifferentiated liposarcoma (DDLPS);
- myxoid liposarcoma (MLPS);
- pleomorphic liposarcoma (PLPS);
- mixed cell liposarcoma (MCLPS), showing features of combined myxoid/ round cell liposarcoma and well-differentiated/dedifferentiated or of myxoid/round cell and pleomorphic liposarcoma).

Each histotype is associated with unique genetic mutations and histologic morphologies, which ultimately impact their behavior. DDLPS and MCLPS are considered high grade tumors whereas low-grade comprises WDLPS, MLPS and round cell subtypes. A MLPS can be considered high grade if more than 5% of tumor cells are round cells.

The prevalence of the different subtypes in primary retroperitoneal liposarcomas is around 50% for WDLPS, from 20% to 37% for DDLPS and less than 3% for the myxoid/round cell type [1–6]. OS at 5 years is 87% for retroperitoneal WDLPS and 41% for DDLPS G3. The cumulative incidence of local relapse at 5 years is 33% for DDLPS G3, 44% for DDLPS G2 and 18% in WDLPS [2].

Histologic subtype has been shown to be the most important predictor of local recurrence and distal metastasis, so that, based on the WHO classification, patients operated on for liposarcoma can be risk-tratified according to histological subtypes [10–16].

8.2.1.1 Well-differentiated Liposarcoma

In WDLPS, the *MDM2* gene, located in 12q14-15, is consistently amplified, usually accompanied by amplification of neighboring genes, such as *SAS*, *CDK4*, and *HMGIC*. This 12q14-15 amplification is not observed in lipomas and its detection may therefore serve to distinguish WDLPS from benign adipose tumors. In contrast to atypical lipomatous tumor, retroperitoneal WDLPS is characterized by a high rate of local recurrence of >40% and an overall mortality >80%.

8.2.1.2 Dedifferentiated Liposarcoma

In DDLPS fluorescence in situ hybridization analysis reveal amplification of the *MDM2* gene also observed in WDLPS [3]. DDLPS is both locally aggressive and has distant metastatic potential. The local recurrence and distant metastasis rates range from 40% to 80% and 15% to 20%, respectively. DDLPS is traditionally conceptualized as a biphasic malignant adipocytic neoplasm that can be: entirely well differentiated; well differentiated with a dedifferentiated component (sometimes more than one in the same tumor); and rarely dedifferentiated without a well differentiated component [12].

Tumors may arise de novo in approximately 90% of cases whilst approximately 10% occur following recurrences from WDLPS. Clinically, there may be a history of a long-standing stable fatty tumor that incurred sudden increase in size. Transformation from WDLPS to DDLPS is thought to occur but the mechanism is not well understood (Fig. 8.1).

Singer et al. reported that 39 of 99 WDLPS patients developed at least one local recurrence, with 32 (83%) recurring as WDLPS and 7 (17%) as high-grade DDLPS. They also reported that after a first WDLPS recurrence, the second recurrence remained WDLPS in 56% and transformed to DDLPS in 44%, suggesting that there is an evolution of mutations with each subsequent recurrence [17].

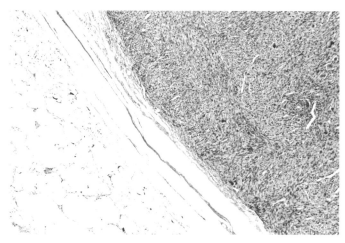

Fig. 8.1 High grade spindle cell sarcoma (dedifferentiated liposarcoma) with evidence of transition to well-differentiated liposarcoma

Besides histologic tumor grading, myogenic differentiation has been shown to be a prognostic factor for DDLPS in the retroperitoneum [18].

8.2.2   Role of Tumor Grade

It is well known that a more aggressive tumor grade is associated with increased risk for recurrence and death [16].

In the largest series of primary RPS that included all histologic subtypes (n=1007), the Trans-Atlantic Retroperitoneal Sarcoma Working Group (TARPSWG) reported that tumor grade was associated with local recurrence, distant metastasis, and overall survival. A subset analysis of this series shows that, among 370 DDLPS stratified by Fédération Nationale des Centres de Lutte Contre le Cancer (FNCLCC) grade, the pattern of failure differs based on the FNCLCC grade of DDLPS. Grade II DDLPS had an 8-year OS of 50%, a local recurrence risk of 50% and distant metastasis risk less than 10%. Grade III DDLPS, on the other hand, had an 8-year OS of 30%, a local recurrence risk of 35%, and a distant metastasis risk of 30% [1].

In studies specific to liposarcoma, Neuhaus et al. reported that high grade of primary RLPS is associated with increased local recurrence (HR=2.48, p=0.035) and worse disease-specific survival (HR=4.14, p=0.005) [19]. In study from the Memorial Sloan-Kettering Cancer Center also focused on all liposarcomas, Linehan et al. reported that for primary RLPS (n=98), the 5-year local RFS rate was 25% for high grade RLPS compared to 49% for low grade RLPS (RR=1.9, p=0.01) [11]. In a larger subsequent study of primary RLPS (n=177) from the Memorial Sloan-Kettering Cancer Center, Singer et al. reported that primary tumor grade was associated with time to local recurrence on univariate analysis but not on multivariate analysis [17]. In a study by Grobmyer et al. higher grade of the first recurrent tumor was associated with worse overall survival compared to lower grade (HR=5.3, p=0.0001) [13]. On the other hand, in a larger series by Park et al., grade of the first local recurrence did not impact the second local RFS in 61 patients who underwent resection of the first local recurrence [20].

8.2.3   Role of Margin Status

Margin status has been extensively investigated as a third factor that contributes to recurrence, even if the association of margins to the oncologic outcomes of RLPS is based on limited data and various definitions of positive margin (microscopic positive v/s gross positive).

In general, however, grossly positive margins are associated with an increased risk for local recurrence whereas microscopically positive resection margins do not necessarily lead to a higher risk of local recurrence [21]. This is predominantly related to a lack of standardization of the sampling protocol to assess surgical margins status. Masses are usually pretty large and difficult to orientate especially relevant to the margins at risk, even in the presence of the operating surgeon. An effort to standardize this process is underway, but the data available so far concerning this are limited and flawed at best.

In order to overcome this limitation most of the series have only separated patients with grossly incomplete (R2) from those with macroscopic complete resections (R0–R1) and of course have shown a worse outcome for patients undergoing R2 resections. However, few series have tried to separate R0 resections from R1 resections and – as expected – results were conflicting.

In essence, the current classification of surgical adequacy is based only on a macroscopic evaluation of the completeness of resection. A joint effort is being made in order to improve it by adding information on the microscopic margin status, but this is still far from being established.

8.3 Management of Recurrent Retroperitoneal Liposarcoma

Resection of recurrent disease has been proven to prolong OS in carefully selected patients, but the potential benefit of resection must be balanced against the associated morbidity and mortality of surgery [1].

The work-up of suspected local recurrence is similar to the one of primary RLPS and requires multidisciplinary evaluation [5, 7, 9, 22–28].

Guidelines for the multidisciplinary management of these patients have been previously reported by the TARPSWG [7] (Tables 8.1 and 8.2).

Sites of recurrence (Figs. 8.2–8.7) are usually categorized as:
(a) locoregional (at the site of the primary RPS or within the ipsilateral retroperitoneum);
(b) multifocal/contralateral retroperitoneum;
(c) both.

Time to disease recurrence is an important factor to consider as it reflects tumor biology and has been shown to correlate with OS.

8.3.1 Preoperative Planning

Initial evaluation of patients with a suspected recurrence requires careful review of prior treatment of their original primary as well as any prior recurrences [1, 11, 20].

Similar to primary RPS, contrast-enhanced computed tomography is critical in evaluating the extent of tumor involvement. Magnetic resonance imaging may be useful in pelvic tumors, while positron-emission tomography is rarely useful.

Table 8.1 Guidelines for the management of recurrent retroperitoneal sarcoma (RPS) in the adult. (adapted from [7])

Multidisciplinary case conference	• Surgical oncologists • Medical oncologists • Radiation oncologists • Pathologists • Radiologists
Imaging	Imaging studies prior to resection of the primary RPS
	Initial postoperative baseline imaging to evaluate prior resection
	CT-CAP – extent and progression of recurrent disease – pattern of relapse (locoregional vs. peritoneal) – rate of progression
	MRI – pelvic tumors or tumors that abut/involve bone or psoas or oblique muscles or vertebral foramen
	PET scan – extent of active abdominal disease
Pathology	Primary tumor reviewed by a specialized pathologist – molecular subtyping
Percutaneous core biopsy	• To provide a definitive diagnosis • To guide selection of preoperative therapies • As part of a translational research program or clinical trial
Patient evaluation	• Symptoms and performance • Previous skin incisions • Renal function and nutritional status
Review of previous treatment	Operative note
	Timing from previous surgery
	Factors that precluded previous macroscopically complete resection
	Previous pathology reports
	Previous surgery should be categorized (1) macroscopically complete (en bloc resection) (2) macroscopically incomplete (gross residual disease as noted on operative report or on immediate postoperative cross-sectional imaging) (3) piecemeal and/or associated with tumor rupture or morcellation
	Previous radiotherapy or systemic therapy

CT-CAP, oral and intravenous contrast-enhanced computed tomography of the chest, abdomen and pelvis; *MRI*, magnetic resonance imaging; *PET*, positron-emission tomography.

A percutaneous biopsy should be recommended in selected cases to confirm the diagnosis as a recurrence may be mistaken for another process such as a radiation-associated sarcoma or to determine the histologic subtype for potential palliative systemic or radiation therapy when the relapse is not resectable or when considering preoperative treatment [1, 5, 11, 22–28].

Table 8.2 Patient selection for surgical resection in retroperitoneal liposarcoma (adapted from [7])

Abdominal recurrence	Isolated locoregional recurrence	Complete gross resection *intent: curative*
	Local recurrence of WDLPS within the field of previous resection(s)	period of observation to space out the interval between operations and to select more favorable candidates
	Multifocal intra-abdominal disease	- very careful approach to patient selection - to avoid complications of progression and to preserve function *intent: palliative*
	Histopathologic subtype	WDLPS favored for re-resection
Distant recurrence	Oligo-metastatic recurrence	metastasectomy
	Synchronous abdominal and distant recurrence	should not be resected consider systemic therapy
Preoperative therapy	Neoadjuvant therapy	cytotoxic and/or targeted systemic therapies in DDLPS
	Preoperative EBRT	if no previous EBRT and isolated recurrence
Postoperative systemic therapy and other locoregional therapies	Prophylactic systemic therapy	no proven role
	Brachytherapy or postoperative EBRT	no proven role
	IORT	evidence is weak
	Intraperitoneal chemotherapy	no proven role
	Regional hyperthermia	no proven role
Treatment of patients not eligible for curative resection	Cytotoxic and/or targeted systemic therapies	subsequent reconsideration of re-section
	Palliative procedures	EBRT R2 resection for symptom control

WDLPS, well-differentiated liposarcoma; *DDLPS*, dedifferentiated liposarcoma; *EBRT*, external beam radiation therapy; *IORT*, intraoperative radiation therapy.

8.3.2 Surgical Technical Principles

In the case of an isolated local recurrence, the surgical principles are superimposable to those for primary RPS and should consider a number of factors: patient history, site, histotype, grading and timing of relapse [20, 27–31].

The purpose of resection is curative and should include en bloc resection of adjacent organs that are directly involved. As is known, surgery in recurrent

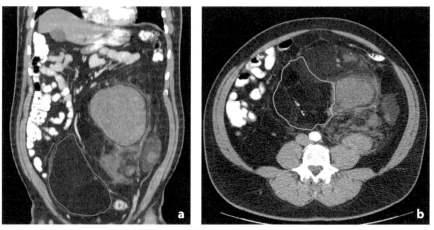

Fig. 8.2 Coronal (**a**) reconstruction and axial (**b**) computed tomography images, showing the left retroperitoneal abdominal mass at diagnosis, with well- differentiated lipidic components (*blue line*) and dedifferentiated solid components (*red line*)

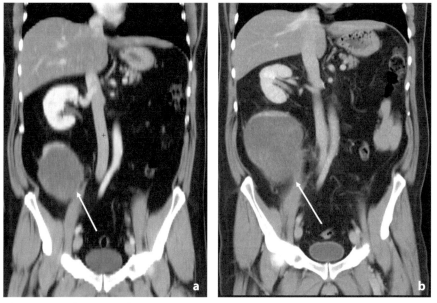

Fig. 8.3 Coronal reconstructions of computed tomography scan after three years (**a**), showing the appearance of a recurrence in the right retroperitoneal space *(white arrow)*, and a growth of the mass after other 6 months of follow-up (**b**)

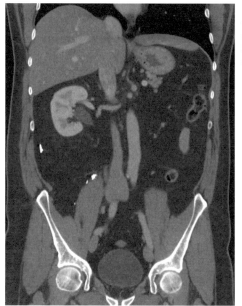

Fig. 8.4 Coronal reconstruction of a computed tomography scan performed after the complete resection of the recurrence, showing the absence of fragments of the lesion

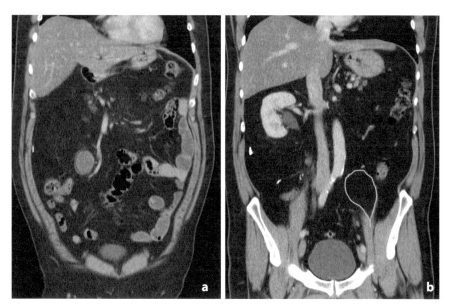

Fig. 8.5 Coronal reconstructions of a computed tomography scan performed after two years from the last surgery performed on the right side, showing a recurrence on the right side (**a**), with a dedifferentiated hyperdense solid mass (*red line*), and a recurrence on the left side (**b**), with well differentiated hypodense lipidic components (*blue line*)

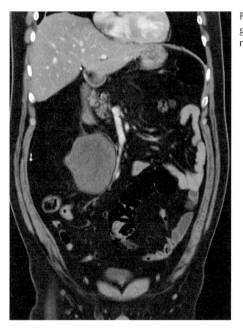

Fig. 8.6 Coronal reconstruction showing the growth of the right solid dedifferentiated recurrence (*red line*)

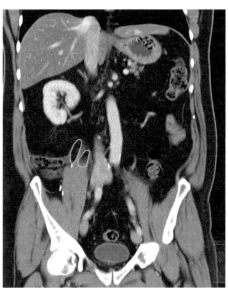

Fig. 8.7 Coronal reconstruction of a computed tomography scan performed a few months after the surgical removal of the recurrence, showing the appearance of a well differentiated recurrence (*blue lines*) along the surface of the right psoas muscle

RLPS can be challenging due to the presence of adhesions, distortion of normal anatomy, and the loss of tissue planes from prior operations.

The TARPSWG [7] performed a subset analysis of those patients who developed recurrence from the original dataset of 1007 patients. Those patients (all histologic subtypes) who underwent surgery for the first local recurrence had improved 5-year OS rates compared to those who did not (43% vs. 11%, p<0.001). The crude cumulative incidence of second local recurrence following resection was 40% at 2 years and 58% at 5 years and the crude cumulative incidence of distant metastasis following resection of first local recurrence was 12% at 2 years and 16% at 5 years [7].

It is well known that the complete resection rate significantly decreases with each subsequent local recurrence. Considering all histotypes, and adapting to the resections of WDLPS and DDLPS, the decline in complete resection rate likely reflects the technical difficulty of multiple abdominal procedures and the aggressive biology of recurrent disease.

In a review of 231 RPS treated at the Memorial Sloan-Kettering Cancer Center, the complete resection rates for primary RPS, first recurrence, second recurrence, and third recurrence were 80%, 57%, 33%, and 14%, respectively [28]. Grobmyer et al. reported similar data in a study of 78 patients. Complete resection rates for first recurrence, second recurrence, and third recurrence were 60%, 39%, and 36%, respectively [13].

8.3.2.1 Timing of resection

The time to first local recurrence and time to surgery for the first local recurrence reflects the biological features of the RLPS. To define the biology of the tumor a period of observation and serial imaging for smaller tumors in asymptomatic patients has been suggested.

Since the probability of long-term disease-free survival is low, an observation period may be helpful in selecting appropriate patients for resection. This is also justified by the evidence, in few retrospective series, that a longer time to recurrence and to surgery is associated with better oncologic outcomes.

In the series from the TARPSWG on management of first recurrent RPS, the median time to local recurrence for 219 patients was 23 months [7]. The majority of patients had liposarcoma (80%). Longer time interval to first local recurrence and surgical resection of first recurrence proved to be predictors of improved OS on multivariable analysis. These data suggest that time to recurrence is important in identifying patients with favorable tumor biological features who will benefit of surgical resection.

In a report specific to locally recurrent liposarcoma, the Memorial Sloan-Kettering Cancer Center reported on 105 patients who had at least one local recurrence following complete resection of a primary RLPS. In this series, 58% of patients had complete resection of their first local recurrent liposarcoma. Local recurrent tumor growth rate was calculated by the size of the tumor divided by the number of months from primary resection to first local recurrence. Tumor size was defined as the maximum cross-sectional dimension for a solitary mass and the sum of all maximal dimensions for multiple masses. The authors observed that after resection of the first local recurrence, the second local RFS was significantly improved for those RLPS patients whose local recurrent tumor growth rate was less than 0.9 cm/month (HR=2.70, $p<0.001$). In addition, the median disease specific survival was longer (100 vs. 21 months) for those who underwent resection and had local recurrent tumor growth rate less than 0.9 cm/month (HR=2.19, p=0.001) [20]. Based on these results, the "1 cm a month rule" became a useful tool to measure the growth rapidity of the tumor, and select patients with a low tumor growth rate, better candidates for surgical resection.

8.3.3   Multifocal Tumors and Sarcomatosis

Multifocal local recurrence can affect 47–57% of patients with a first local recurrence [30]. Resection is typically reserved for palliation in symptomatic patients and presents a significant technical challenge.

Tseng et al. reported that patients with unifocal RLPS (WDLPS and DDLPS) developed multifocal local recurrence in 57% of cases. Of these patients, about 20% developed tumors distant from the original surgical field. Interestingly, a prior piecemeal/R2 resection or multiorgan surgery did not predict multifocal or outside the field of resection recurrence [12].

Van Dalen et al. reported that out of 77 patients who underwent complete resection of RPS, 42% of cases developed a local recurrence. The majority of these patients (62%) were liposarcoma, with nearly half of them with multifocal disease. The 5-year OS rates were 58% and 20% for unifocal and multifocal disease (p=0.01) [9]. Conversely, Grobmyer et al. reported that multifocality did not appear to affect OS on multivariate analysis [13].

With the aim of defining the difference between multifocal recurrence and peritoneal sarcomatosis, Anaya et al. reported that 42% of patients with multifocal disease had RLPS. In a multivariable analysis, they found that multifocal disease >7 tumors was associated with worse OS and that incomplete debulking and chemotherapy were not associated with improved OS. The authors suggested that since unifocal and multifocal ≤7 tumors had better prognosis than multifocal >7 tumors, a cut-off of 7 tumors defines peritoneal sarcomatosis [31].

There are few series that report the use of cytoreduction with or without intraperitoneal chemotherapy in the management of recurrent RLPS. Most studies include multiple sarcoma histologic subtypes such as liposarcoma and gastrointestinal stromal tumor. In a study from the Istituto Nazionale Tumori in Milan, 37 patients with sarcomatosis were treated with cytoreductive surgery and hyperthermic intraperitoneal chemotherapy (HIPEC). Patients with sarcomatosis secondary to RLPS (n=13) had the best OS (median, 34 months) with a local RFS of 12 months. However, all 13 patients developed peritoneal relapse [32]. The MD Anderson Cancer Center reported the results of two phase

I trials of cytoreduction and HIPEC (n=28 patients) and concluded that HIPEC was associated with significant toxicity and limited clinical benefit [33].

8.3.4 Unresectable Disease

The role of surgical debulking for unresectable RLPS was reviewed by Shibata et al. in 55 patients. Of the 26 patients who presented with locally recurrent unresectable disease, 19 underwent incomplete resection of the disease. The authors reported that median OS was superior for those whose median time to recurrence was greater than 24 months (median OS: 26 vs. 10 months; $p=0.02$). The authors concluded that incomplete surgical resection can offer some survival benefit in selected patients [34].

Resection of distant metastases has been shown to be associated with significantly improved disease-specific survival, however, resection should be avoided in patients with concomitant local recurrence and distant metastases.

For patients with unresectable disease, systemic therapy for WDLPS/DDLPS has been evaluated. In a retrospective review of 208 patients with unresectable or metastatic liposarcoma (161 with RLPS) treated at 11 institutions, Italiano et al. reported that the objective response rate was higher for anthracycline-containing regimens. There was no difference in objective response observed between WDLPS and DDLPS (13% vs. 12%, $p=0.9$). The median OS was 33.5 months for WDLPS and 13.9 months for DDLPS [35].

8.4 Radiation

The role of adjuvant radiation for recurrent or residual RLPS is even more controversial than in primary disease. To date, data on the use of radiotherapy in recurrent RLPS come from retrospective series on different histotypes and treatment methods. Patients who received radiotherapy for recurrence are those who did not receive it previously, mainly retroperitoneal DDLPS.

In the series reported by the TARPSWG, patients with first locally recurrent disease had no improvement in outcome associated with radiation and chemotherapy for the recurrence in the whole series as well as in RLPS subgroup [7].

Hamilton et al. studied the outcomes of patients with recurrent or residual RPS. The 5-year local re-recurrence rate and OS rates were 56% and 57%, respectively, which was not significantly different from studies not employing radiation as an adjuvant to surgical resection of recurrences [25].

If delivered preoperatively, electron-beam radiation therapy has the advantage that the recurrent or residual disease can be targeted in situ.

8.5   Systemic Treatment

Systemic therapy for locally recurrent RLPS that is resectable is generally not recommended, particularly for WDLPS, as little evidence supports the use of systemic therapy for primary and recurrent RLPS.

In a retrospective review of 88 liposarcoma patients (38 with RLPS) who received chemotherapy at the Royal Marsden Hospital, the objective response rate was 0% for WDLPS and 25% for DDLPS. The progression-free survival for WDLPS and DDLPS was 11 and 2 months, respectively [36].

Novel and more effective systemic therapies are required to meet the needs of these patients. Targeted therapy could offer chances when a specific biologic feature is detected. However, the relative rarity of these entities and the diverse molecular and genetic characteristics of each subtype curb the development of new therapies [37, 38]. Recently the Cancer Genome Atlas (TCGA) sarcoma analysis focused on six major adult soft tissue sarcomas including DDLPS [39]. To identify oncogenic drivers and potential therapeutic targets they integrated genome analyses of mRNA, miRNA, DNA sequence, methylation and copy number variation. In 50 cases of DDLPS they observed recurrent copy number gains and recurrent deletions, mainly in *ATRX* whose expression may be required for response to *CDK4* inhibitors [39]. *ATRX* could represent a biomarker for anti CDK4 trials. In the same way *Jun* amplification could become a target.

Another field that has been explored is the potential feasibility of immunotherapy in this disease. The evaluation of intratumoral immune response (PD-1 and PD-L1 expression, tumor-infiltrating lymphocytes and the tumor microenvironment) can offer new opportunities [40, 41]. In the study SARC028, pembrolizumab showed encouraging activity in patients with undifferentiated pleomorphic sarcoma or DDLPS [42].

In conclusion, RLPS encompasses a number of different subtypes with distinct biology and clinical behavior. Recent advances in better understanding the subtype specific biology could identify new therapeutic targets.

References

1.   Gronchi A, Strauss DC, Miceli R et al (2016) Variability in patterns of recurrence after resection of primary retroperitoneal sarcoma (RPS): a report on 1007 patients from the multi-institutional collaborative RPS working group. Ann Surg 263(5):1002–1009

2. Gronchi A, Miceli R, Allard MA et al (2015) Personalizing the approach to retroperitoneal soft tissue sarcoma: histology-specific patterns of failure and postrelapse outcome after primary extended resection. Ann Surg Oncol 22(5):1447–1454
3. Tan MC, Brennan MF, Kuk D et al (2016) Histology-based classification predicts pattern of recurrence and improves risk stratification in primary retroperitoneal sarcoma. Ann Surg 263(3):593–600
4. Bonvalot S, Rivoire M, Castaing M et al (2009) Primary retroperitoneal sarcomas: a multivariate analysis of surgical factors associated with local control. J Clin Oncol 27(1):31–37
5. Gronchi A, Lo Vullo S, Fiore M et al (2009) Aggressive surgical policies in a retrospectively reviewed single-institution case series of retroperitoneal soft tissue sarcoma patients. J Clin Oncol 27(1):24–30
6. Lehnert T, Cardona S, Hinz U et al (2009) Primary and locally recurrent retroperitoneal soft-tissue sarcoma: local control and survival. Eur J Surg Oncol 35(9):986–993
7. Trans-Atlantic RPS Working Group (2016) Management of recurrent retroperitoneal sarcoma (RPS) in the adult: a consensus approach from the Trans-Atlantic RPS Working Group. Ann Sur Oncol 23(11):3531–3540
8. Gronchi A, Casali PG, Fiore M et al (2004) Retroperitoneal soft tissue sarcomas: patterns of recurrence in 167 patients treated at a single institution. Cancer 100(11):2448–2455
9. van Dalen T, Hoekstra HJ, van Geel AN et al; Dutch Soft Tissue Sarcoma Group (2001) Locoregional recurrence of retroperitoneal soft tissue sarcoma: second chance of cure for selected patients. Eur J Surg Oncol 27(6):564–568
10. Fletcher CDM, Bridge JA, Hogendoorn PCW, Mertens F (2013) WHO classification of tumors of soft tissue and bone, 4th edn. IARC Press, Lyon
11. Linehan DC, Lewis JJ, Leung D, Brennan MF (2000) Influence of biologic factors and anatomic site in completely resected liposarcoma. J Clin Oncol 18(8):1637–1643
12. Tseng WW, Madewell JE, Wei W et al (2014) Locoregional disease patterns in well-differentiated and dedifferentiated retroperitoneal liposarcoma: implications for the extent of resection? Ann Surg Oncol 21(7):2136–2143
13. Grobmyer SR, Wilson JP, Apel B et al (2010) Recurrent retroperitoneal sarcoma: impact of biology and therapy on outcomes. J Am Coll Surg 210(5):602–608
14. De Sanctis R, Giordano L, Colombo C et al (2017) Long-term follow-up and post-relapse outcome of patients with localized retroperitoneal sarcoma treated in the Italian Sarcoma Group-Soft Tissue Sarcoma (ISG-STS) Protocol 0303. Ann Surg Oncol 24(13):3872–3879
15. Dei Tos AP (2014) Liposarcomas: diagnostic pitfalls and new insights. Histopathology 64(1):38–52
16. Yang JY, Kong SH, Ahn HS et al (2015) Prognostic factors for reoperation of recurrent retroperitoneal sarcoma: the role of clinicopathological factors other than histologic grade. J Surg Oncol 111(2):165–172
17. Singer S, Antonescu CR, Riedel E, Brennan MF (2003) Histologic subtype and margin of resection predict pattern of recurrence and survival for retroperitoneal liposarcoma. Ann Surg 238(3):358–370; discussion 370–371
18. Gronchi A, Collini P, Miceli R et al (2015) Myogenic differentiation and histologic grading are major prognostic determinants in retroperitoneal liposarcoma. Am J Surg Pathol 39(3):383–393
19 Neuhaus SJ, Barry P, Clark MA et al (2005) Surgical management of primary and recurrent retroperitoneal liposarcoma. Br J Surg 92(2):246–252
20 Park JO, Qin LX, Prete FP et al (2009) Predicting outcome by growth rate of locally recurrent retroperitoneal liposarcoma: the one centimeter per month rule. Ann Surg 250(6):977–982
21. Stahl JM, Corso CD, Park HS et al (2017) The effect of microscopic margin status on survival in adult retroperitoneal soft tissue sarcomas. Eur J Surg Oncol 43(1):168–174

22. Gyorki DE, Brennan MF (2014) Management of recurrent retroperitoneal sarcoma. J Surg Oncol 109(1):53–59
23. Hassan I, Park SZ, Donohue JH et al (2004) Operative management of primary retroperitoneal sarcomas: a reappraisal of an institutional experience. Ann Surg 239(2):244–250
24. Lochan R, French JJ, Manas DM (2011) Surgery for retroperitoneal soft tissue sarcomas: aggressive re-resection of recurrent disease is possible. Ann R Coll Surg Engl 93(1):39–43
25. Hamilton TD, Cannell AJ, Kim M et al (2017) Results of resection for recurrent or residual retroperitoneal sarcoma after failed primary treatment. Ann Surg Oncol 24(1):211–218
26. MacNeill AJ, Miceli R, Strauss DC et al (2017) Post-relapse outcomes after primary extended resection of retroperitoneal sarcoma: a report from the Trans-Atlantic RPS Working Group. Cancer 123(11):1971–1978
27. Gronchi A, Miceli R, Colombo C et al (2012) Frontline extended surgery is associated with improved survival in retroperitoneal low- to intermediate-grade soft tissue sarcomas. Ann Oncol 23(4):1067–1073
28   Lewis JJ, Leung D, Woodruff JM, Brennan MF (1998) Retroperitoneal soft-tissue sarcoma: analysis of 500 patients treated and followed at a single institution. Ann Surg 228(3):355–365
29. Fairweather M, Gonzales RJ, Strauss D, Raut CP (2018) Current principles of surgery for retroperitoneal sarcomas. J Surg Oncol 117(1):33–41
30. Bagaria SP, Gabriel E, Mann GN (2018) Multiply recurrent retroperitoneal liposarcoma. J Surg Oncol 117(1):62–68
31   Anaya DA, Lahat G, Liu J et al (2009) Multifocality in retroperitoneal sarcoma: a prognostic factor critical to surgical decision-making. Ann Surg 249(1):137–142
32. Baratti D, Pennacchioli E, Kusamura S et al (2010) Peritoneal sarcomatosis: is there a subset of patients who may benefit from cytoreductive surgery and hyperthermic intraperitoneal chemotherapy. Ann Surg Oncol 17(12):3220–3228
33   Lim SJ, Cormier JN, Feig BW et al (2007) Toxicity and outcomes associated with surgical cytoreduction and hyperthermic intraperitoneal chemotherapy (HIPEC) for patients with sarcomatosis. Ann Surg Oncol 14(8):2309–2318
34. Shibata D, Lewis JJ, Leung DH, Brennan MF (2001) Is there a role for incomplete resection in the management of retroperitoneal liposarcomas? J Am Coll Surg 193(4):373–379
35. Italiano A, Toulmonde M, Cioffi A et al (2012) Advanced well-differentiated/dedifferentiated liposarcomas: role of chemotherapy and survival. Ann Oncol 23(6):1601–1607
36. Jones RL, Fisher C, Al-Muderis O, Judson IR (2005) Differential sensitivity of liposarcoma subtypes to chemotherapy. Eur J Cancer 41(18):2853–2860
37. Ben Salha I, Zaidi S, Noujaim J et al (2016) Rare aggressive behavior of MDM2-amplified retroperitoneal dedifferentiated liposarcoma, with brain, lung and subcutaneous metastases. Rare Tumors 8(3):6282
38. Patel RB, Li T, Liao Z, Jaldeepbhai JA et al (2017) Recent translational research into targeted therapy for liposarcoma. Stem Cell Investig 4:21
39. Cancer Genome Atlas Research Network (2017) Comprehensive and integrated genomic characterization of adult soft tissue sarcomas. Cell 171(4):950–965
40. Kovatcheva M, Liu DD, Dickson MA et al (2015) MDM2 turnover and expression of ATRX determine the choice between quiescence and senescence in response to CDK4 inhibition. Oncotarget 6(10):8226–8243
41. Ricciotti RW, Baraff AJ, Jour G et al (2017) High amplification levels of MDM2 and CDK4 correlate with poor outcome in patients with dedifferentiated liposarcoma: a cytogenomic microarray analysis of 47 cases. Cancer Genet 218–219:69–80
42. Tawbi HA, Burgess M, Bolejack V et al (2017) Pembrolizumab in advanced soft-tissue sarcoma and bone sarcoma (SARC028): a multicentre, two-cohort, single-arm, open-label, phase 2 trial. Lancet Oncol 18(11):1493–1501

Management of Other Recurrent Retroperitoneal Sarcomas

Marco Rastrelli, Saveria Tropea, and Carlo Riccardo Rossi

9.1 Introduction

The anatomic peculiarities of the retroperitoneum (lack of boundaries to allow true compartmental surgical resection with safe margins, the proximity of vital structures and visceral organs, and asymptomatic growth of huge masses) and the biological heterogeneity of sarcomas lead to a challenging management of retroperitoneal soft tissue sarcoma (RPS). As a result of the limit to achieve wide resection margins, local recurrences of RPS are not rare [1–13]. Furthermore, different histological subtypes and grades have different patterns and timing of recurrence, with biological behavior spanning a broad spectrum from no metastatic potential, to a propensity for local recurrence to a mainly distant relapse [2, 13, 14]. RPS other than liposarcoma are very rare and the main histological subtypes are: leiomyosarcoma (LMS), solitary fibrous tumor (SFT), malignant peripheral nerve sheath tumor (MPNST), synovial sarcoma (SS), undifferentiated pleomorphic sarcoma (UPS), Despite the rich heterogeneity, LMS and SFT are the most frequent [2–4, 10, 11, 13, 15–17].

Generally, local recurrence rates are higher in patients with high/intermediate grade tumors compared with those with low-grade tumors. Recurrent RPS is associated with a worse prognosis. In fact, many patients with recurrent disease are candidates for re-resection but reoperation may be associated with considerable morbidity and mortality. In detail, redo surgery has been shown to increase survival and provide symptomatic relief in some patients. In fact, local recurrence and/or its treatment is one of the most common causes of death from local recurrent RPS. However, tumor biology, despite the differences in

M. Rastrelli (✉)
Surgical Oncology Unit, Veneto Institute of Oncology IOV-IRCCS
Padua, Italy
e-mail: marco.rastrelli@iov.veneto.it

V. Quagliuolo, A. Gronchi (Eds), *Current Treatment of Retroperitoneal Sarcomas*,
Updates in Surgery
DOI: 10.1007/978-88-470-3980-3_9, © Springer-Verlag Italia 2019

histologic subtype, and tumor grade as well as macroscopic completeness of surgical resection remain the major determinants of long-term outcomes, even if these prognostic factors tend to play a lesser role in determining long-term survival over the course of subsequent reoperations [2, 5, 6, 13–15, 17–19]. Moreover, primary and recurrent RPS other than liposarcoma, especially LMS, display a significant systemic risk. Metastatic RPS includes both systemic disease and multifocal intra-abdominal disease or sarcomatosis. Despite multimodal treatment, outcomes for metastatic RPS are poor with median overall survival (OS) of 16 months [13, 20].

All these aspects lead to a great deal of management controversy and the necessity of a tailored treatment for each case. Several studies have analyzed the pattern of recurrence and outcomes of patients with recurrent RPS. However, most of these reports consist of small retrospective studies with limited follow-up, and variable results and patient outcomes. In order to guide sarcoma specialists in the management of patients with recurrent RPS the Trans-Atlantic Retroperitoneal Sarcoma Working Group (TARPSWG) recently published a consensus document [2–13].

9.2   Pretreatment Assessment

Patients affected by RPS should be discussed at multidisciplinary meetings attended by surgical oncologists, medical oncologists, radiation oncologists, pathologists and radiologists, all specialized in soft tissue sarcoma. The operative report of first surgery should be reviewed and the nature of previous surgery should be categorized as macroscopically complete, macroscopically incomplete and piecemeal and/or associated with tumor rupture or morcellation. Also, timing from previous surgery and details of any previously administered radiotherapy or systemic therapy should be noted [2].

9.2.1   Imaging

First, it is necessary to review all relevant imaging studies performed before primary sarcoma resection and the initial postoperative baseline imaging to establish the completeness of resection. Once the extension of surgery has been verified, contrast-enhanced computed tomography (CT) of the chest, abdomen and pelvis should be performed to assess current extent of local and distant disease and compared to all prior imaging to determine the progression rate of recurrent disease and tumor invasion into adjacent organs or critical structures [2, 21, 22].

Abdominal magnetic resonance imaging (MRI) may be a useful diagnostic modality in patients with intravenous contrast allergy or other serious contraindications to CT. MRI is also indicated in selected cases, where the anatomic relationship of disease to specific neurovascular structures is not clear, for operative planning of pelvic tumors and RPS that involves bone or psoas or oblique muscles and vertebral foramen. MRI is also the gold standard of imaging to characterize suspected brain and soft tissue metastases [2, 21, 23].

Positron emission tomography (PET) is rarely indicated and it may be required if the extent of active abdominal disease is difficult to evaluate and there is uncertainty about different growth features in multifocal lesions. It may also be useful in differentiating metastatic disease from other benign affections and to evaluate medical treatment response [2, 24, 25].

9.2.2 Pathology

Previous pathology reports and any tissue slides/blocks from the primary resection should be obtained and reviewed by pathologists with expertise in soft tissue tumors [2].

In cases of local relapse, if disease is multifocal and/or associated with distant metastases with a radiographic pattern typical of recurrence, confirmation with tissue sampling is not required. However, especially when radiographic appearance is less characteristic or in the absence of distant metastases, percutaneous core biopsy confirmation of local recurrence, obtained under image guidance, may represent a good approach to provide a definitive diagnosis and to exclude a series of other disorders that can be easily mistaken for recurrence of the primary RPS (e.g., desmoid fibromatosis, radiation-associated osteosarcoma, lymphoma, metastasis from another primary malignancy). In fact, second surgery is often challenging, with a considerable morbidity rate, and it should not be performed without due cause. However, it may also be necessary to guide the selection of preoperative therapies and as a part of a translational research programs [2, 26].

Concerning distant metastases, if lung and liver lesions are radiographically suggestive of disease, in the context of a histological confirmed primary RPS, it is not necessary to perform another biopsy. However, if these lesions are radiological atypical or in the context of a known second tumor or a hereditary syndrome, a biopsy is recommended to guide future treatments. For subcutaneous or soft tissue lesions suspicious for metastases, biopsy should also be considered [26].

9.2.3 Patient Selection for Resection

The possibility of definitive cure after recurrence is low and therefore a multidisciplinary evaluation is necessary to carefully consider the potential morbidity of second surgery in the single patient. For this purpose, the patient's current performance status and symptoms should be recorded, and renal function and nutritional status should be assessed. Finally, the decision to proceed to a surgical approach is multifactorial and often nuanced [2].

9.3   Clinical Management of Recurrent Retroperitoneal Sarcomas

9.3.1   Preoperative Therapy

Neoadjuvant radiotherapy should be considered, especially if no previous radiotherapy has been administered and the local recurrence is isolated. However, its value in improving disease control has not been well defined and toxicity may be significant in the setting of previous resection.

For patients affected by high grade local recurrent RPS (especially in the case of LMS, UPS, SFT and SS) with a short disease-free interval and when resection is associated with considerable morbidity, neoadjuvant systemic therapies could downsize recurrent disease and thus improve resectability and may also facilitate assessment of tumor biology and prognosis [2].

9.3.2   Treatment of Abdominal Recurrence

The TARPSWG guidelines, in the case of isolated locoregional recurrence, especially if the previous surgery was incomplete, recommended a second curative and complete resection. Regarding surgical technique, to date, the second operation is not intended to remove adherent organs, if not directly infiltrated. Otherwise, surgical resection should be aimed simply at achieving macroscopic resection, including surrounding organs only when overtly infiltrated. Substantial issues make second surgical treatment more difficult than the primitive. Specifically, loss of the original planes and distortion of anatomical relationships may increase the difficulty of determining the extent of disease and thus the optimal extent of resection. The use of intraoperative frozen section on marginal tissues as a guide to extent of resection is generally not advised but, in some specific scenarios, such as LMS of a major vein, frozen section analysis of a vascular margin may be useful if additional tissue at a relevant site can be removed. Moreover, in this setting accidental injuries of important structures are not uncommon. So, as already mentioned, it is important to carefully consider the potential morbidity of second surgery in the single patient [2, 13, 17].

Instead, a history of previous piecemeal resection/tumor rupture indicates a strong potential for multifocal peritoneal recurrence and curative intent surgery is not indicated. In fact, multifocal intra-abdominal disease is difficult to resect completely and it will almost certainly recur with the result of a poor prognosis. Surgery could be indicated in case of symptomatic disease to relieve symptoms (gastrointestinal occlusion, bleeding…). At any rate, resections should be aimed at avoiding complications of progression and preserving function, taking into account that incomplete resection confers no survival benefit and can lead to significant morbidity [2, 10, 27, 28].

After resection, patients should be followed up with regular clinical evaluation and cross-sectional imaging every 3–6 months, given the high risk for further relapse [2, 6, 17].

In selected patients, who are not eligible for curative resection, radiotherapy may be of palliative benefit with control of pain related to nerve compression or infiltration. In the same cases, systemic therapies may improve and prolong quality of life and, if a significant response is detected, a second resection can be reconsidered [2].

9.3.3 Postoperative Systemic Therapy and Other Locoregional Therapies

After complete resection of recurrent RPS, there is no evidence of benefit for adjuvant systemic therapy, radiotherapy or brachytherapy. Intraoperative radiotherapy (IORT) may be considered after resection but the evidence of benefit is weak. Intraperitoneal chemotherapy has no proven value but it may be considered for highly selected patients and histologies (LMS) within the context of clinical trials. In the case of multifocal intraperitoneal sarcoma, the results of debulking surgery and intraperitoneal chemotherapy have been poor with high morbidity. Regional hyperthermia is of no proven value [2, 29–36].

9.3.4 Management of Distant Recurrence

Selected patients with limited oligo-metastatic recurrence of RPS, which applies especially to LMS, may have prolonged survival following metastasectomy. Patients should be considered eligible for metastasectomy only if the primary tumor was completely resected and if they show a favorable biology in terms of low volume disease, a disease-free interval of at least 12 months and a confirmed response to chemotherapy or a prolonged stable disease ($\geq$6 months) on systemic therapy. Following the diagnosis of potentially resectable metastases, a period of "wait and see" may be established to ascertain disease biology. Furthermore, in patients candidate to pulmonary resection, lung function should be optimized before surgery and patients should undergo preoperative pulmonary function testing before planned resection. If the surgeon has appropriate expertise in

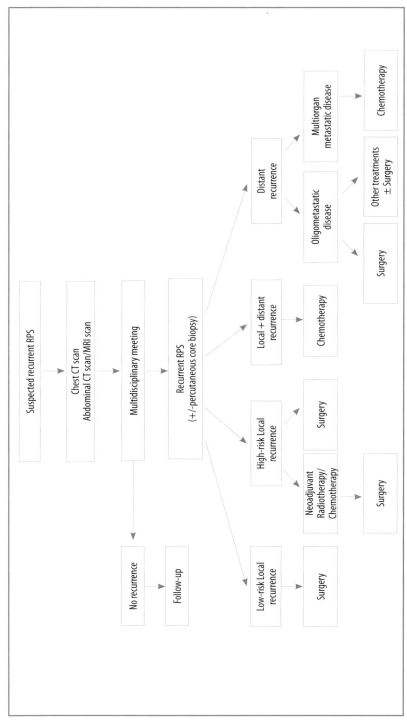

Fig. 9.1 Management of other recurrent retroperitoneal sarcomas (RPS)

the minimally invasive technique, this surgical approach can also be taken into account [2, 26]. In recent years, other local therapies, such as radiofrequency ablation, microwave ablation and stereotactic body radiotherapy, have been shown to achieve similar rates of disease control for hepatic and pulmonary recurrence; thus, they are considered acceptable alternatives with lower complication rates. This applies all the more for patients with compromised pulmonary function who are not eligible for surgical resection. Moreover, these treatment modalities can be combined with surgery to obtain complete disease eradication. However, with regard to survival outcomes, there is no evidence that patients have prolonged survival because of the treatment itself rather than a consistent selection of patients with a favorable biology. Furthermore, available literature data consist of relatively small and retrospective mixed series of bone and soft tissue sarcoma with the limit of the inclusion of multiple histologic subtypes and anatomic sites of origin (retroperitoneal vs. extremity/trunk) [2, 37–48].

Regarding synchronous abdominal and distant recurrence or synchronous metastases, they should not be generally resected and the patient should be destined to systemic therapy. In fact, surgical resection has not been associated with improved survival. However, in selected patients, the concomitance of pulmonary and extrapulmonary metastases is not an absolute contraindication to curative treatment and occasionally prolonged survival can be observed with complete resection of multiorgan disease [2, 26].

Surveillance with imaging every 3–6 months is needed after resection of metastatic disease, because many patients will develop recurrent metastases. Repeated surgery may only be considered in cases of favorable biology and long disease-free interval; on the contrary, high grade histology, high tumor volume, and short disease-free intervals are associated with poor prognosis and further surgery is not recommended (Fig. 9.1) [26].

9.4   Recurrent Leiomyosarcoma

According to the TARPSWG, leiomyosarcoma displayed a significant systemic risk (>50%). The extended primary approach optimized local control (95% at 5 years) but it could not prevent distant spread, in comparison to other RPS (especially liposarcoma), which have a predominant local pattern of recurrence. To date, the few local recurrences of LMS have been treated with a second surgery. Interestingly, LMS had a better outcome after distant metastasis compared to all other histotypes and this could be related to the availability of multiple lines of chemotherapy and several potentially active drugs such as dacarbazine, anthracycline, gemcitabine, trabectedin and, more recently, pazopanib [2, 13, 14, 17]. These data are supported by the TARPSWG report on postrelapse outcomes after primary extended resection of RPS. Specifically, TARPSWG results revealed that of the 408 patients who experienced disease recurrences after resection of primary RPS, the initial site of recurrence was local for only 219 patients, distant for only 146 patients and both local and distant for 43 patients. Among these, the percentage of patients with a histological diagnosis of LMS was 7%, 53% and 23%, respectively. Moreover, at multivariate Cox model analysis, it was found that, in patients who developed distant metastases only, significant independent prognostic factors of improved OS were a longer time to distant metastases and LMS histology. Furthermore, resection of distant metastases was a significant predictor of improved disease-specific survival [13].

Another retrospective study confirmed that, following resection, retroperitoneal LMS spread more frequently at distant sites than local ones and, in particular, the most common sites are the lungs followed by the liver, skin or soft tissue, distant lymph nodes, bone, pancreas, brain and spinal cord. Moreover, it found that surgery for recurrences was associated with improved OS and that location (distant or local) or multifocality was not related to OS. However, this study also demonstrated that the second recurrence rate was high and that the only positive prognostic factor that predicted progression-free survival was a longer disease-free interval (>12 months) [49].

9.5 Recurrent Solitary Fibrous Tumor

Solitary fibrous tumor represents a very rare disease and few studies are available on the natural history of this tumor. It showed an indolent course, although an aggressive variant exists. Few local recurrences and distant metastases were observed at 5 years. Nevertheless, a longer follow-up may be advisable to define its relapse rate because late local and distant metastases have been reported. Surgery of the few recurrences may be discussed in a multidisciplinary sarcoma meeting [13, 17].

9.6 Other Variants

Other variants of retroperitoneal sarcoma such as MPNST, SS, UPS and desmoplastic small round cell tumor (DSCRT) are very rare. Management of local and distant recurrence should be remanded to multidisciplinary sarcoma teams, as explained above [2, 13, 17].

References

1. Trans-Atlantic RPS Working Group (2015) Management of primary retroperitoneal sarcoma (RPS) in the adult: a consensus approach from the Trans-Atlantic RPS Working Group. Ann Surg Oncol 22(1):256–263
2. Trans-Atlantic RPS Working Group (2016) Management of recurrent retroperitoneal sarcoma (RPS) in the adult: a consensus approach from the Trans-Atlantic RPS Working Group. Ann Surg Oncol 23(11):3531–3540
3. Callegaro D, Miceli R, Mariani L et al (2017) Soft tissue sarcoma nomograms and their incorporation into practice. Cancer 123(15):2802–2820
4. Raut CP, Miceli R, Strauss DC et al (2016) External validation of a multi-institutional retroperitoneal sarcoma nomogram. Cancer 122(9):1417–1424
5. Gronchi A, Casali PG, Fiore M et al (2004) Retroperitoneal soft tissue sarcomas: patterns of recurrence in 167 patients treated at a single institution. Cancer 100(11):2448–2455
6. Grobmyer SR, Wilson JP, Apel B et al (2010) Recurrent retroperitoneal sarcoma: impact of biology and therapy on outcomes. J Am Coll Surg 210(5):602–608, 608–610
7. Koenig AM, Reeh M, Burdelski CM et al (2012) Long-term results of primary and secondary resections in patients with retroperitoneal soft tissue sarcoma. Langenbecks Arch Surg 397(8):1251–1259
8. Bonvalot S, Miceli R, Berselli M et al (2010) Aggressive surgery in retroperitoneal soft tissue sarcoma carried out at high-volume centers is safe and is associated with improved local control. Ann Surg Oncol 17(6):1507–1514
9. Bonvalot S, Raut CP, Pollock RE et al (2012) Technical considerations in surgery for retroperitoneal sarcomas: position paper from E-Surge, a master class in sarcoma surgery, and EORTC-STBSG. Ann Surg Oncol 19(9):2981–2991
10. Lochan R, French JJ, Manas DM (2011) Surgery for retroperitoneal soft tissue sarcomas: aggressive re-resection of recurrent disease is possible. Ann R Coll Surg Engl 93(1):39–43
11. Neuhaus SJ, Barry P, Clark MA et al (2005) Surgical management of primary and recurrent retroperitoneal liposarcoma. Br J Surg 92(2):246–252
12. van Dalen T, Hoekstra HJ, van Geel AN et al; Dutch Soft Tissue Sarcoma Group (2001) Locoregional recurrence of retroperitoneal soft tissue sarcoma: second chance of cure for selected patients. Eur J Surg Oncol 27(6):564–568
13. MacNeill AJ, Miceli R, Strauss DC et al (2017) Post-relapse outcomes after primary extended resection of retroperitoneal sarcoma: a report from the Trans-Atlantic RPS Working Group. Cancer 123(11):1971–1978
14. Gronchi A, Strauss DC, Miceli R et al (2016) Variability in patterns of recurrence after resection of primary retroperitoneal sarcoma (RPS): a report on 1007 patients from the Multi-institutional Collaborative RPS Working Group. Ann Surg 263(5):1002–1009
15. Gyorki DE, Brennan MF (2014) Management of recurrent retroperitoneal sarcoma. J Surg Oncol 109(1):53–59
16. Chiappa A, Zbar AP, Bertani E et al (2006) Primary and recurrent retroperitoneal soft tissue sarcoma: prognostic factors affecting survival. J Surg Oncol 93(6):456–463
17. Gronchi A, Miceli R, Allard MA et al (2015) Personalizing the approach to retroperitoneal soft tissue sarcoma: histology-specific patterns of failure and postrelapse outcome after primary extended resection. Ann Surg Oncol 22(5):1447–1454
18. Anaya DA, Lahat G, Wang X et al (2010) Postoperative nomogram for survival of patients with retroperitoneal sarcoma treated with curative intent. Ann Oncol 21(2):397–402
19. Nathan H, Raut CP, Thornton K et al (2009) Predictors of survival after resection of retroperitoneal sarcoma: a population-based analysis and critical appraisal of the AJCC staging system. Ann Surg 250(6):970–976
20. Toulmonde M, Bonvalot S, Ray-Coquard I et al; French Sarcoma Group (2014) Retroperitoneal sarcomas: patterns of care in advanced stages, prognostic factors and focus on main histological subtypes: a multicenter analysis of the French Sarcoma Group. Ann Oncol 25(3):730–734

21. Morosi C, Stacchiotti S, Marchianò A et al (2014) Correlation between radiological assessment and histopathological diagnosis in retroperitoneal tumors: analysis of 291 consecutive patients at a tertiary reference sarcoma center. Eur J Surg Oncol 40(12):1662–1670

22. Tzeng CW, Smith JK, Heslin MJ (2007) Soft tissue sarcoma: preoperative and postoperative imaging for staging. Surg Oncol Clin N Am 16(2):389–402

23. Shiraev T, Pasricha SS, Choong P et al (2013) Retroperitoneal sarcomas: a review of disease spectrum, radiological features, characterisation and management. J Med Imaging Radiat Oncol 57(6):687–700

24. Niccoli-Asabella A, Altini C, Notaristefano A et al (2013) A retrospective study comparing contrast-enhanced computed tomography with 18F-FDG-PET/CT in the early follow-up of patients with retroperitoneal sarcomas. Nucl Med Commun 34(1):32–39

25. Alford S, Choong P, Chander S et al (2012) Value of PET scan in patients with retroperitoneal sarcoma treated with preoperative radiotherapy. Eur J Surg Oncol 38(2):176–180

26. Trans-Atlantic Retroperitoneal Sarcoma Working Group (TARPSWG) (2018) Management of metastatic retroperitoneal sarcoma: a consensus approach from the Trans-Atlantic Retroperitoneal Sarcoma Working Group (TARPSWG). Ann Oncol 29(4):857–871

27. Anaya DA, Lahat G, Liu J et al (2009) Multifocality in retroperitoneal sarcoma: a prognostic factor critical to surgical decision-making. Ann Surg 249(1):137–142

28. Yang JY, Kong SH, Ahn HS et al (2015) Prognostic factors for reoperation of recurrent retroperitoneal sarcoma: the role of clinicopathological factors other than histologic grade. J Surg Oncol 111(2):165–172

29. Woll PJ, Reichardt P, Le Cesne A et al; EORTC Soft Tissue and Bone Sarcoma Group and the NCIC Clinical Trials Group Sarcoma Disease Site Committee (2012) Adjuvant chemotherapy with doxorubicin, ifosfamide, and lenograstim for resected soft-tissue sarcoma (EORTC 62931): a multicentre randomised controlled trial. Lancet Oncol 13(10):1045–1054

30. Smith MJ, Ridgway PF, Catton CN et al (2014) Combined management of retroperitoneal sarcoma with dose intensification radiotherapy and resection: long-term results of a prospective trial. Radiother Oncol 110(1):165–171

31. Tseng WH, Martinez SR, Do L et al (2011) Lack of survival benefit following adjuvant radiation in patients with retroperitoneal sarcoma: a SEER analysis. J Surg Res 168(2):e173–e180

32. Roeder F, Ulrich A, Habl G et al (2014) Clinical phase I/II trial to investigate preoperative dose-escalated intensity-modulated radiation therapy (IMRT) and intraoperative radiation therapy (IORT) in patients with retroperitoneal soft tissue sarcoma: interim analysis. BMC Cancer 14:617

33. Hayes-Jordan A, Green HL, Lin H et al (2014) Complete cytoreduction and HIPEC improves survival in desmoplastic small round cell tumor. Ann Surg Oncol 21(1):220–224

34. Hayes-Jordan A (2015) Cytoreductive surgery followed by hyperthermic intraperitoneal chemotherapy in DSRCT: progress and pitfalls. Curr Oncol Rep 17(8):38

35. Sugarbaker P, Ihemelandu C, Bijelic L (2016) Cytoreductive surgery and HIPEC as a treatment option for laparoscopic resection of uterine leiomyosarcoma with morcellation: early results. Ann Surg Oncol 23(5):1501–1507

36. Angele MK, Albertsmeier M, Prix NJ et al (2014) Effectiveness of regional hyperthermia with chemotherapy for high-risk retroperitoneal and abdominal soft-tissue sarcoma after complete surgical resection: a subgroup analysis of a randomized phase-III multicenter study. Ann Surg 260(5):749–754

37. Nakamura T, Matsumine A, Yamakado K et al (2009) Lung radiofrequency ablation in patients with pulmonary metastases from musculoskeletal sarcomas [corrected]. Cancer 115(16):3774–3781

38. Palussière J, Marcet B, Descat E et al (2011) Lung tumors treated with percutaneous radiofrequency ablation: computed tomography imaging follow-up. Cardiovasc Intervent Radiol 34(5):989–997

39. Dhakal S, Corbin KS, Milano MT et al (2012) Stereotactic body radiotherapy for pulmonary metastases from soft-tissue sarcomas: excellent local lesion control and improved patient survival. Int J Radiat Oncol Biol Phys 82(2):940–945
40. Koelblinger C, Strauss S, Gillams A (2014) Outcome after radiofrequency ablation of sarcoma lung metastases. Cardiovasc Intervent Radiol 37(1):147–153
41. Falk AT, Moureau-Zabotto L, Ouali M et al; Groupe Sarcome Francais-Groupe d'Etude des Tumeurs Osseuses (2015) Effect on survival of local ablative treatment of metastases from sarcomas: a study of the French sarcoma group. Clin Oncol (R Coll Radiol) 27(1):48–55
42. Savina M, Le Cesne A, Blay JY et al (2017) Patterns of care and outcomes of patients with METAstatic soft tissue SARComa in a real-life setting: the METASARC observational study. BMC Med 15(1):78
43. Frakulli R, Salvi F, Balestrini D et al (2015) Stereotactic radiotherapy in the treatment of lung metastases from bone and soft-tissue sarcomas. Anticancer Res 35(10):5581–5586
44. Navarria P, Ascolese AM, Cozzi L et al (2015) Stereotactic body radiation therapy for lung metastases from soft tissue sarcoma. Eur J Cancer 51(5):668–674
45. Brudvik KW, Patel SH, Roland CL et al (2015) Survival after resection of gastrointestinal stromal tumor and sarcoma liver metastases in 146 patients. J Gastrointest Surg 19(8):1476–1483
46. Jones RL, McCall J, Adam A et al (2010) Radiofrequency ablation is a feasible therapeutic option in the multi modality management of sarcoma. Eur J Surg Oncol 36(5):477–482
47. Baumann BC, Nagda SN, Kolker JD et al (2016) Efficacy and safety of stereotactic body radiation therapy for the treatment of pulmonary metastases from sarcoma: a potential alternative to resection. J Surg Oncol 114(1):65–69
48. Pawlik TM, Vauthey JN, Abdalla EK et al (2006) Results of a single-center experience with resection and ablation for sarcoma metastatic to the liver. Arch Surg 141(6):537–543; discussion 543–544
49. Ikoma N, Torres KE, Lin HY et al (2017) Recurrence patterns of retroperitoneal leiomyosarcoma and impact of salvage surgery. J Surg Oncol 116(3):313–319

The Role of Radiation Therapy in the Treatment of Retroperitoneal Sarcomas

10

Antonino De Paoli, Federico Navarria, Elisa Palazzari,
Piera Navarria, and Claudia Sangalli

10.1 Introduction

Retroperitoneal soft tissue sarcomas (RPS) are rare tumors, accounting for 10–15% of all soft tissue sarcomas. The estimated annual incidence is 1–2 cases per million inhabitants [1]. Because of the anatomical peculiarities, the retroperitoneal location still faces many challenges. Typically, these tumors are large in size and they may involve vital structures within the abdominal cavity at the time of diagnosis.

Surgery remains the only potentially curative therapy for these malignancies. However, the results in terms of disease control and survival are still disappointing in most published series [2]. Even though the data have improved in recently reported experiences with more aggressive multivisceral surgery, wide surgical margins are not achievable in most cases and local recurrences may be still a problem [3–5].

Looking at the evidence for adding radiation therapy (RT) to surgery, well established for the extremity soft tissue sarcomas, data are still lacking in RPS and the results of the European Organisation for Research and Treatment of Cancer - Soft Tissue and Bone Sarcoma Group (EORTC-STBSG) trial addressing this issue are awaited (NCT01344018). Therefore, a close collaboration between surgeons and radiation oncologists, and discussion in dedicated multidisciplinary tumor boards are essential in the decision-making process to possibly combine the two treatment modalities on an individualized basis.

At present, patterns of clinical practice on the use of RT in the treatment of RPS are widely variable. In a population-based study on 2348 cases, Porter

A. De Paoli (✉)
Radiation Oncology Department, IRCCS CRO-Aviano, National Cancer Institute
Aviano, Pordenone, Italy
e-mail: adepaoli@cro.it

V. Quagliuolo, A. Gronchi (Eds), *Current Treatment of Retroperitoneal Sarcomas*,
Updates in Surgery
DOI: 10.1007/978-88-470-3980-3_10, © Springer-Verlag Italia 2019

et al. [6] in 2006 reported that outside clinical trials, only 25.9% of patients received RT and 85.5% of them were treated with postoperative RT (postop RT). These data were confirmed in a Surveillance, Epidemiology, and End Results (SEER) analysis recently reported by Bates et al. in 2015 [7]; of 480 patients, 30% received RT and all were treated with postop RT. More recently, in a multi-institutional series of 1007 patients reported by Gronchi et al. in 2016 [8], 32% received RT and, interestingly, 72% of them were treated with preoperative RT (preop RT). Thus, although not consistently, an interest in the use of preop RT has been emerging in more recent years.

10.2   Timing of Treatment: Preoperative or Postoperative Radiation Therapy

Both preop and postop RT are options in the treatment of soft tissue sarcomas and debate continues regarding the optimal timing relative to surgery. For extremity sarcomas, randomized trials and large retrospective database analysis have been reported. Although with a significant higher incidence of early local complications after preop RT, better long-term results and limb function have been reported and preop RT is widely considered the preferred treatment option [9, 10].

This question is of particular interest also in the treatment of RPS, as they arise in a critical anatomical site. On this issue, the retrospective National Cancer Data Base (NCDB) study recently reported by Nussbaum et al. [11] is of particular interest. The study involved 9068 patients with RPS and was performed using a case-control, propensity score-matched principles to minimize selection biases. In this series, 563 patients received preop RT, 2215 postop RT and 6290 surgery alone. Most patients who received preop RT were treated in dedicated-sarcoma centers, at least in more recent years. Both preop RT (HR 0.70) and postop RT (HR 0.78) were significantly associated with improved overall survival compared with surgery alone. The series is retrospective, and many data are lacking in the NCDB, including events other than deaths. The propensity score matched comparison is sound, but it can fail to detect differences in the selection of patients for RT, as paradoxically RT may have been used in the better cases, simply because the treatment was feasible. However, the series is large and the advantage in survival intriguing, supporting the hypothesis that the administration of RT may play a role, especially for patients affected by RPS, the natural history of which is predominantly characterized by a local risk.

No randomized data are available so far. Thus, no definitive conclusions can be drawn both regarding the role and the optimal timing of RT in the management of RPS.

10.3   Postoperative Radiation Therapy

The high risk of local recurrence after surgery prompted the addition of postop RT in the treatment of patients with RPS. The rationale for this approach was based on extrapolation of data from phase III trials of adjuvant postop RT for patients with sarcomas of the extremities [12, 13]. The hypothesis was that RT could have a potential role in the treatment of RPS, provided it may be administered with an acceptable toxicity. Only few series have been reported with postop RT in RPS [14–20]. These series were all retrospective and included a limited number of patients who underwent either complete or partial resection. In addition, a wide range of radiation doses were used (14–62 Gy) depending on target volumes and the radiation tolerance of the normal critical abdominal structures. No survival benefit was reported in these series compared to historical controls with surgery alone, but a possible impact on local control was noted in patients treated with higher doses of radiation when complete resection proved feasible. Two analyses of the SEER database on postop RT for RPS were reported. A first series on 1350 patients reported by Tzeng et al. [20] in 2011 showed no survival benefit. The second was published by Bates et al. [7] in 2015 and reported a benefit in high grade disease. Importantly, a marked toxicity was of concern and severe late complications (infection, hemorrhage, malabsorption, bowel obstruction) were reported in 19–40% of patients in the more recently published series; 19% of complications at 4 years of follow-up after a median dose of 50 Gy (14–62 Gy) were reported by Le Pechoux et al. [16], 25% after a dose up to 60 Gy were reported by Pezner et al. [17], and 40% at 3.5 years after 50 Gy were reported by Zlotecki et al. [15]. These data suggested a possible benefit of RT in the treatment of RPS when adequate doses of radiation can be safely delivered. However, this objective is difficult to obtain in the postoperative setting because of the limited dose tolerance of multiple critical structures in this anatomical site and the radiation doses typically used for extremities are often unfeasible.

10.4   Preoperative Radiation Therapy

Given the limitations of postop RT and the emerging preference for preop RT in extremity sarcomas, an interest in preop RT has emerged also for RPS. Recently, an international expert panel was convened to develop a consensus on RT guidelines for RPS [21]. A consensus was reached that preop RT should be preferred to postop RT for several reasons including: the tumor mass allows the displacement of normal structures outside the RT volume, thereby reducing the risk of complications; target volume definition is much more accurate when the tumor is still in place; potential radiobiological advantage of improved

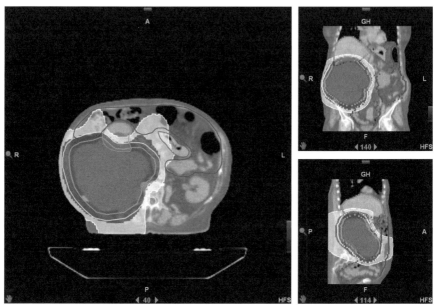

Fig. 10.1 Preoperative IMRT-IGRT with tomotherapy for retroperitoneal sarcoma (CRO Aviano)

oxygenation of tumor cells in the preoperative setting; decreased risk of tumor implantation at the time of surgical resection; possible reduction in tumor size with thickening of the pseudocapsule, which may allow better dissection planes at surgical resection; and finally, extrapolating data from the extremity sarcoma studies, the possible equivalence of 50 Gy in the preop setting with 60–66 Gy in the postop one.

The panel recommendations include details on patient preparation, planning-computed tomography (CT) acquisition and target volume delineation. The gross tumor volume (GTV) should be contoured on the 4D-CT scan (to incorporate motion assessment) for upper retroperitoneal sarcomas. An expansion of GTV by 2 to 2.5 cm in cephalocaudal direction and 1.5 to 2 cm radially to create the clinical target volume (CTV) is suggested. Advanced treatment techniques such as intensity modulated RT (IMRT) are recommended for the superior dose conformality with improved sparing of organs at risk. Because of documented interfractional RPS tumor movement, a daily image-guide radiation therapy (IGRT) is indicated (cone-beam CT or megavolt CT). The preoperative dose of 50–50.4 Gy in 25–28 daily fractions of 1.8–2 Gy is recommended. An example of IMRT-IGRT with tomotherapy in the treatment of RPS is reported in Figure 10.1.

Only few studies have investigated the role of preop RT in RPS (Table 10.1). Tzeng et al. [22] reported a preoperative dose escalation program with IMRT in a series of 16 patients; 45 Gy were given to entire tumor volume and a simultaneous boost up to 57.5 Gy included the area of tumor considered to be at high risk for

Table 10.1 Preoperative radiation followed by surgery with or without intraoperative radiation therapy (selected series)

Study	n/IOERT	5-year LC (%)	5-year OS (%)	IOERT/EBRT (Gy)	Plan	Toxicity (%)
Pawlik et al. [26]	72/34	52	61	15–25/45	3D RT	[4 preop deaths]
Petersen et al. [24]	87/87	59	47	12.5–15/48.6	NA	PN: 36 (10 severe)
Gieschen et al. [23]	37/20	59	50	15/45	2-field	PN: 5.4; GI: 5.4
Tzeng et al. [22]	16/0	80 (2 years)	94 (2 years)	12.5 (EBRT)/57.5	IMRT	GI: 37.5 (mild)
Zlotecki et al. [15]	15/0	66	NA	NA/50.4, 1.2 BID	3D RT	GI: 36 (enteritis)

IOERT, intraoperative electron beam radiation therapy; *LC,* local control; *OS,* overall survival; *EBRT,* external beam radiation therapy; *BID,* twice-a-day; *3D-RT,* three-dimensional radiation therapy; *IMRT,* intensity modulated radiation therapy; *PN,* peripheral neuropathy; *GI,* gastrointestinal; NA, not applicable.

positive margins after surgery, typically the area of tumor adherent the posterior abdominal wall, vertebral bodies and major abdominal vessels. The results were encouraging in terms of efficacy and safety and this approach is gaining a growing interest. Other preop RT series reported dose escalation with intraoperative electron beam radiation therapy (IOERT). Gieschen et al. [23] reported data on 37 patients treated with preop RT 45 Gy, 20 of them received IOERT with 10–15 Gy. Treatment was well tolerated with interesting results in local control. These data were reproduced in selected series at the Mayo Clinic by Petersen et al. [24] and at the MD Anderson Cancer Center by Pisters et al. [25].

Although preop RT, with or without dose escalation, proved to be safe and effective, its impact on treatment of RPS awaits the results of the recently completed EORTC-STBSG trial.

10.5   Combined Preoperative Chemotherapy and Radiotherapy

In an attempt to improve the sensitivity of sarcoma to preop RT and provide a systemic adjuvant treatment, a combined preop chemotherapy and RT approach has been investigated in resectable, primary or recurrent RPS. Only two prospective studies have been reported.

The first was a phase I trial promoted at the MD Anderson Cancer Center and published by Pisters et al. [25] in 2003. The investigators treated 35 patients with resectable RPS with preoperative doxorubicin, 4 mg/m²/d, and concurrent RT with dose escalation from 18 to 50.4 Gy followed by surgery and IOERT. Treatment was tolerated fairly well; only two patients experienced grade 3–4 toxicity, but six patients (17%) had disease progression during therapy that precluded the planned surgery. Of note, 90% of operated patients had complete (R0–R1) resection. Long-term results were then reported by Pawlik et al. [26] in 2006 in an update of two institutional experiences on a prospective-based protocol with preop RT including data from the MD Anderson Cancer Center and the University of Toronto. The 5-year local control and survival rates were 60% and 61%, respectively.

The second study was a phase I-II collaborative trial promoted by the Italian Sarcoma Group and initially reported by Gronchi et al. [27] in 2014. Patients received 3 cycles of high-dose continuous-infusional ifosfamide with a daily dose of 1 g/m² for 14 consecutive days, every 4 weeks, and concurrent RT of 50.4 Gy. A total of 83 patients were accrued and 79 underwent surgery, macroscopically complete (R0–R1) in 88% of patients. IOERT was given in selected cases. Four patients (5%) progressed before surgery. Local and distant recurrences at 5 years occurred in 37% and 26%, respectively. Although the results were encouraging, this combination was feasible in two-thirds of patients and hematological toxicity was the main cause of treatment interruption. Long-term follow-up and postrelapse outcomes have been recently reported by De Sanctis et al. [28] in 2017. The 7-year recurrence-free survival and overall survival were 46.6% and 63.2%, respectively, and the cumulative incidence of local recurrence and distant metastasis were 37.4% and 20%, respectively. Most local recurrences were in-field and the prognosis of relapsed patients was poor.

These experiences support the possible efficacy of preoperative concurrent chemo-radiotherapy in RPS as an available option for patients on an individualized basis choice.

10.6   Intraoperative Radiation Therapy

Intraoperative electron-beam radiation therapy (IOERT) is a treatment modality of some interest in the treatment of RPS. When combined with external-beam irradiation, IOERT may allow dose escalation to the tumor bed after resection in a particularly favorable treatment time (Fig. 10.2). IOERT combined with preop or postop RT has been evaluated at many institutions in the treatment of RPS. However, the addition of IOERT 10–15 Gy to surgery and postoperative external-beam RT of 45–50.4 Gy resulted in high local control rates in one study only [29]. In the phase III trial conducted at the National Cancer Institute, a significant advantage in local control was reported for patients treated with IOERT (20 Gy) and postop EBRT (35–40 Gy) compared to EBRT (50–55 Gy)

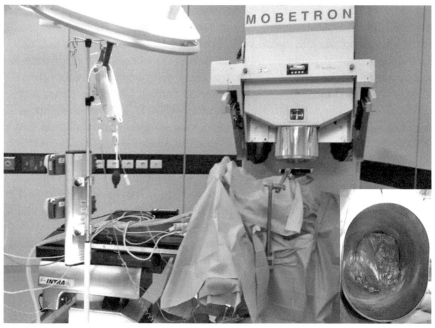

Fig. 10.2 IOERT administered with a mobile linear accelerator in the operating room (CRO Aviano)

alone (20% vs. 80% in-field local recurrences, respectively). Of note overall survival was similar in both groups and severe small bowel complications were less frequent in patients who underwent IOERT + EBRT. On the contrary, peripheral neuropathy rates were higher in the IOERT group [30]. Other retrospective studies confirmed the feasibility of IOERT plus postoperative EBRT with better neurological tolerance with IOERT dose <12.5 Gy [24, 31].

More recently, some interest has emerged in the combination of IOERT or perioperative brachytherapy to preop RT for the management of RPS. Results of some selected series are reported in Table 10.1. There is no strong evidence that the addition of IOERT to preop RT is effective, while it is known to add to morbidities, in particular with perioperative brachytherapy. The reported rates of local control were encouraging. Morbidity from treatment was considered acceptable, even though up to 20% of IOERT-treated patients experienced treatment-related complications.

10.7   Proton Beam Therapy

Protons allow the delivery of higher and more focused radiation dose to tumor with less exposure to the surrounding tissues [32]. Because of the usual large size of RPS at presentation, they are often in close proximity to significant volumes of radiation-sensitive abdominal structures such as the bowel, stomach, liver, kidney, ureters and spinal cord. For these reasons, among all soft tissue sarcomas in adult patients, RPS are those who may benefit the most from the use of protons in preop RT [32]. Treatment planning comparisons for preop RT demonstrated that intensity modulated proton therapy (IMPT) achieves a dose conformality comparable to more conventional IMRT with photons, but with the additional benefit of lower integral dose (i.e., total body radiation dose). The bowel median volume receiving 15 Gy or more (V15) was 16.4% for IMPT, 52.2% for IMRT and 66% for 3D-CRT and the median volume receiving 45 Gy or more (V45) was 6.3% for IMPT, 4.7% for IMRT and 15.6% for 3D-conformal radiotherapy when a standard dose of 50.4 Gy to planning target volume was planned [33, 34]. The ability to selectively increase the dose in the target volume with either IMRT or IMPT offers the possibility of dose escalation to selected, high risk areas of the target such as posterior abdominal wall, major abdominal vessels and vertebral bodies where it is difficult to achieve an adequate surgical margin at surgery [22, 35]. This dose painting approach in preop RT with IMRT or IMPT may avoid the risk of late toxicity reported in dose escalation programs with IOERT (or allows more moderate IOERT dose), such as neuropathy, because of lower radiation fraction size. This issue of selective dose escalation with IMRT or IMPT is currently being investigated in a multicentric phase I-II study at the Massachusetts General Hospital. The study includes two separate IMPT and IMRT cohorts. Dose escalation to 63 Gy was safely achieved in the IMPT group and was recently reported by DeLaney et al. [36]. The phase II study is currently ongoing with the 63 Gy dose level (Fig. 10.3).

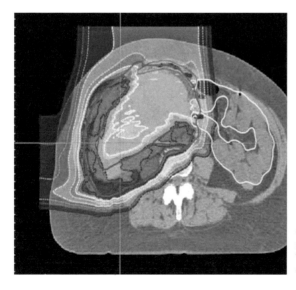

Fig. 10.3 Preoperative radiation dose escalation to high risk area with IMPT. By courtesy of T.F. DeLaney, Massachusetts General Hospital, Boston, USA

10.8   Conclusions

Because of the rarity and the need for expertise in the multidisciplinary management of sarcomas, and RPS in particular, referral to dedicated centers of all patients with confirmed or suspected RPS is recommended [21]. At present, the role of RT in the treatment of RPS remains controversial. Although postop RT has been associated with lower local recurrence rates in some retrospective series, this approach is associated with substantial toxicity and has been abandoned. Preop RT is emerging as the preferred approach for the encouraging local control rates and treatment tolerance. However, its role has not been proven, and data from EORTC-STBSG randomized trial comparing surgery alone to preop RT followed by surgery are awaited. The addition of dose escalation programs with new techniques such as IOERT or proton therapy, or treatment intensification with concurrent chemoradiotherapy, currently remains of investigational interest and should continue to be further evaluated in clinical studies.

References

1. Siegel RL, Miller KD, Jemal A (2015) Cancer statistics, 2015. CA Cancer J Clin 65(1):5–29
2. Tseng WW, Seo HJ, Pollock RE, Gronchi A (2018) Historical perspectives and future directions in the surgical management of retroperitoneal sarcoma. J Surg Oncol 117(1): 7–11
3. Gronchi A, Lo Vullo S, Fiore M et al (2009) Aggressive surgical policies in a retrospectively reviewed single-institution case series of retroperitoneal soft tissue sarcoma patients. J Clin Oncol 27(1):24–30
4. Bonvalot S, Rivoire M, Castaing M et al (2009) Primary retroperitoneal sarcomas: a multivariate analysis of surgical factors associated with local control. J Clin Oncol 27(1):31–37
5. Stojadinovic A, Leung DH, Hoos A et al (2002) Analysis of the prognostic significance of microscopic margins in 2,084 localized primary adult soft tissue sarcomas. Ann Surg 235(3):424–434
6. Porter GA, Baxter NN, Pisters PW (2006) Retroperitoneal sarcoma: a population-based analysis of epidemiology, surgery, and radiotherapy. Cancer 106(7):1610–1616
7. Bates JE, Dhakal S, Mazloom A, Constine LS (2018) The benefit of adjuvant radiotherapy in high-grade nonmetastatic retroperitoneal soft tissue sarcoma: a SEER analysis. Am J Clin Oncol 41(3):274–279
8. Gronchi A, Strauss DC, Miceli R et al (2016) Variability in patterns of recurrence after resection of primary retroperitoneal sarcoma (RPS): a report on 1007 patients from the multi-institutional collaborative RPS working group. Ann Surg 263(5):1002–1009
9. O'Sullivan B, Davis AM, Turcotte R et al (2002) Preoperative versus postoperative radiotherapy in soft-tissue sarcoma of the limbs: a randomised trial. Lancet 359(9325):2235–2241
10. Sampath S, Schultheiss TE, Hitchcock YJ et al (2011) Preoperative versus postoperative radiotherapy in soft-tissue sarcoma: multi-institutional analysis of 821 patients. Int J Radiat Oncol Biol Phys 81(2): 498–505

11. Nussbaum DP, Rushing CN, Lane WO et al (2016) Preoperative or postoperative radiotherapy versus surgery alone for retroperitoneal sarcoma: a case-control, propensity score-matched analysis of a nationwide clinical oncology database. Lancet Oncol 17(7):966–975

12. Yang JC, Chang AE, Baker AR et al (1998) Randomized prospective study of the benefit of adjuvant radiation therapy in the treatment of soft tissue sarcomas of the extremities. J Clin Oncol 16(1):197–203

13. Pisters PW, Harrison LB, Leung DH et al (1996) Long-term results of a prospective randomized trial of adjuvant brachytherapy in soft tissue sarcoma. J Clin Oncol 14(3): 859–868

14. Bishop AJ, Zagars GK, Torres KE et al (2015) Combined modality management of retroperitoneal sarcomas: a single-institution series of 121 patients. Int J Radiat Oncol Biol Phys 93(1):158–165

15. Zlotecki RA, Katz TS, Morris CG et al (2005) Adjuvant radiation therapy for resectable retroperitoneal soft tissue sarcoma: the University of Florida experience. Am J Clin Oncol 28(3):310–316

16. Le Péchoux C, Musat E, Baey C et al (2013) Should adjuvant radiotherapy be administered in addition to front-line aggressive surgery (FAS) in patients with primary retroperitoneal sarcoma? Ann Oncol 24(3):832–837

17. Pezner RD, Liu A, Chen YJ et al (2011) Full-dose adjuvant postoperative radiation therapy for retroperitoneal sarcomas. Am J Clin Oncol 34(5):511–516

18. Gilbeau L, Kantor G, Stoeckle E et al (2002) Surgical resection and radiotherapy for primary retroperitoneal soft tissue sarcoma. Radiother Oncol 65(3):137–143

19. Trovik LH, Ovrebo K, Almquist M et al (2014) Adjuvant radiotherapy in retroperitoneal sarcomas. A Scandinavian Sarcoma Group study of 97 patients. Acta Oncol 53(9): 1165–1172

20. Tseng WH, Martinez SR, Do L et al (2011) Lack of survival benefit following adjuvant radiation in patients with retroperitoneal sarcoma: a SEER analysis. J Surg Res 168(2): e173–e180

21. Baldini EH, Wang D, Haas RL et al (2015) Treatment guidelines for preoperative radiation therapy for retroperitoneal sarcoma: preliminary consensus of an international expert panel. Int J Radiat Oncol Biol Phys 92(3):602–612

22. Tzeng CW, Fiveash JB, Popple RA et al (2006) Preoperative radiation therapy with selective dose escalation to the margin at risk for retroperitoneal sarcoma. Cancer 107(2):371–379

23. Gieschen HL, Spiro IJ, Suit HD et al (2001) Long-term results of intraoperative electron beam radiotherapy for primary and recurrent retroperitoneal soft tissue sarcoma. Int J Radiat Oncol Biol Phys 50(1):127–131

24. Petersen IA, Haddock MG, Donohue JH et al (2002) Use of intraoperative electron beam radiotherapy in the management of retroperitoneal soft tissue sarcomas. Int J Radiat Oncol Biol Phys 52(2):469–475

25. Pisters PW, Ballo MT, Fenstermacher MJ et al (2003) Phase I trial of preoperative concurrent doxorubicin and radiation therapy, surgical resection, and intraoperative electron-beam radiation therapy for patients with localized retroperitoneal sarcoma. J Clin Oncol 21(16):3092–3097

26. Pawlik TM, Pisters PW, Mikula L et al (2006) Long-term results of two prospective trials of preoperative external beam radiotherapy for localized intermediate- or high-grade retroperitoneal soft tissue sarcoma. Ann Surg Oncol 13(4):508–517

27. Gronchi A, De Paoli A, Dani C et al (2014) Preoperative chemo-radiation therapy for localised retroperitoneal sarcoma: a phase I-II study from the Italian Sarcoma Group. Eur J Cancer 50(4):784–792

28. De Sanctis R, Giordano L, Colombo C et al (2017) Long-term follow-up and post-relapse outcome of patients with localized retroperitoneal sarcoma treated in the Italian Sarcoma Group-Soft Tissue Sarcoma (ISG-STS) Protocol 0303. Ann Surg Oncol 24(13):3872–3879

29. Roeder F, Alldinger I, Uhl M et al (2018) Intraoperative electron radiation therapy in retroperitoneal sarcoma. Int J Radiat Oncol Biol Phys 100(2):516–527
30. Sindelar WF, Kinsella TJ, Chen PW et al (1993) Intraoperative radiotherapy in retroperitoneal sarcomas. Final results of a prospective, randomized, clinical trial. Arch Surg 128(4):402–410
31. Calvo FA, Azinovic I, Martinez R et al (1995) Intraoperative radiotherapy for the treatment of soft tissue sarcomas of central anatomical sites. Radiat Oncol Invest 3(2):90–96
32. DeLaney TF, Haas RLM (2016) Innovative radiotherapy of sarcoma: proton beam radiation. Eur J Cancer 62:112–123
33. Swanson EL, Indelicato DJ, Louis D et al (2012) Comparison of three-dimensional (3D) conformal proton radiotherapy (RT), 3D conformal photon RT, and intensity-modulated RT for retroperitoneal and intra-abdominal sarcomas. Int J Radiat Oncol Biol Phys 83(5):1549–1557
34. Chung CS, Trofimov A, Adams J et al (2006) A comparison of 3D conformal proton therapy, intensity modulated proton therapy, and intensity modulated photon therapy for retroperitoneal sarcoma. Int J Radiat Oncol Biol Phys 66 (3 Suppl):S116
35. Yoon SS, Chen YL, Kirsch DG et al (2010) Proton-beam, intensity-modulated, and/or intraoperative electron radiation therapy combined with aggressive anterior surgical resection for retroperitoneal sarcomas. Ann Surg Oncol 17(6):1515–1529
36. DeLaney TF, Chen YL, Baldini EH et al (2017) Phase 1 trial of preoperative image guided intensity modulated proton radiation therapy with simultaneously integrated boost to the high risk margin for retroperitoneal sarcomas. Adv Radiat Oncol 2(1):85–93

Medical Therapy in Retroperitoneal Sarcomas

11

Giovanni Grignani, Roberta Sanfilippo, and Alexia F. Bertuzzi

11.1 Introduction

The rarity and heterogeneity of soft tissue sarcomas (STS) make clinical decision-making in the management of retroperitoneal sarcomas (RPS) always a challenging task [1]. This is particularly true for medical treatment wherein most of the available data are derived from either collections of sarcomas arising in both the limbs and retroperitoneum or retrospective series [2, 3]. Thus, it is of utmost importance to precisely define the clinical setting in which medical therapy is proposed and the intrinsic limitations regarding the strength of evidence underlying the chosen drug/s. Indeed, the role of chemotherapy, still the main tool in the medical treatment of RPS, is not well defined. The lack of consistent evidence in overall survival mandates a careful weighing of the potential benefit against the relevant toxicity associated with these treatments.

Consistently, a dedicated tumor board may be the only appropriate context to assess the role of medical treatment in the frame of a multidisciplinary approach [4]. Therefore, taking for granted that the decision must always be multidisciplinary, we will present the available medical options according to the following categories: localized disease (preoperative and postoperative therapy), local relapse, synchronous or metachronous metastatic disease.

Finally, and despite the fact that almost any sarcoma histotype may affect the retroperitoneum, we will focus on the most frequent forms [5]:

- well-differentiated liposarcoma (WDLPS);
- dedifferentiated liposarcoma (DDLPS);
- leiomyosarcoma (LMS);
- undifferentiated pleomorphic sarcoma (UPS);

G. Grignani (✉)
Department of Medical Oncology, Candiolo Cancer Institute - FPO IRCCS
Candiolo, Turin, Italy
e-mail: giovanni.grignani@ircc.it

V. Quagliuolo, A. Gronchi (Eds), *Current Treatment of Retroperitoneal Sarcomas,*
Updates in Surgery
DOI: 10.1007/978-88-470-3980-3_11, © Springer-Verlag Italia 2019

- solitary fibrous tumor (SFT);
- malignant peripheral nerve sheath tumor (MPNST).

Indeed, histotype affects not only medical choices but the whole treatment strategy even more so after doxorubicin-based chemotherapy. This is even more important in rarer histologies, such as malignant perivascular epithelioid cell neoplasms (so-called PEComas) or the Ewing family of tumors that need to be addressed with different drugs [6].

11.2   General Principles of Medical Treatment

Doxorubicin is the cornerstone of chemotherapy in STS. The largest randomized trial performed in advanced STS by the European Organisation for Research and Treatment of Cancer (EORTC) showed that the combination of doxorubicin and ifosfamide was superior to doxorubicin alone in terms of progression-free survival (PFS) (7.4 vs. 4.6 months, $p=0.003$), overall response rate (ORR) (26% vs. 14%, $p=0.0006$), but not in overall survival (OS) (14.3 vs. 12.8 months, $p=0.076$) [7]. More recently, another randomized phase III trial failed to show that the combination of gemcitabine and docetaxel was superior to doxorubicin in terms of PFS (23.7 vs. 23.3 weeks, $p=0.06$), ORR (20% vs. 19%) and OS (67.3 vs. 76.3 weeks, $p=0.41$) [8]. Therefore, doxorubicin remains the treatment of reference in non-resectable settings regardless of the fact that these data were related to patients mostly affected by limb STS. Another major limitation of these trials is the pooling of STS as if this group of tumors was a single disease. On the contrary, plenty of evidence stands against this simplification especially in the advanced setting, where both retrospective and prospective studies have consistently demonstrated that the opposite is true in what is known as histology-driven chemotherapy [9]. Indeed, ifosfamide is more active in synovial sarcoma compared to LMS; pazopanib is not deemed to be efficacious in liposarcoma (LPS); eribulin showed a sharply greater efficacy in LPS compared to LMS [10–12]. A noteworthy exception is the combination of doxorubicin and the monoclonal antibody anti-PDGFR-α olaratumab. In a small phase I/II trial, the combination of doxorubicin-olaratumab prolonged OS in significantly (26.5 vs. 14.7 months, $p=0.0003$) [13]. While awaiting the final results of the ANNOUNCE study, a large randomized phase III trial, this promising OS advantage led to the conditional approval of this combination by both the European Medicines Agency (EMA) and the Food and Drug Administration (FDA) making this combination the first one to have shown a clear improvement in OS. Hence, anthracycline is still the treatment of reference and any decision on combination chemotherapy should take into account the multimodality strategy planned for that individual patient based on performance status, symptoms, histotype, grading, tumor presentation/extension (local and distant disease), resectability, and radiotherapy. A practical tool to make patient assessment more objective is the nomogram proposed and validated by the Trans-Atlantic Retroperitoneal Sarcoma Working Group (TARPSWG) [14]. Here we will briefly summarize a few general considerations regarding the role of medical treatment. Given the overall modest expected activity of chemotherapy in STS (ORR in the range of 20–30%), and the pivotal role of surgery, medical treatment can be considered in the neoadjuvant setting to improve involvement of adjacent organs (e.g., superior mesenteric artery) [15, 16]. One further advantage of delivering chemotherapy before surgery may also be the fact that nephrectomy is often required and therefore ifosfamide use is more challenging afterwards. Another issue to bear in mind is both the different chemotherapy sensitivity and relative risk of recurrence according to histotype [17]. For instance, LMS entails a higher risk of distant recurrence compared to SFT. However, if deemed necessary by the tumor board, histotype is a clue to a stronger rationale on the use/avoidance of chemotherapy in each specific histotype.

Finally, in some patients, RPS is widely spread in the abdominal cavity already at diagnosis. In this context, as in ovarian cancer, the role of maximal cytoreduction has been advocated followed by hyperthermic intraperitoneal chemotherapy (HIPEC). Once again there is a paucity of data that greatly limits the possibility to draw definitive conclusions. Overall, no OS benefit has ever been shown and its use should be strongly discouraged outside a dedicated clinical trial that should take place only in centers with a solid experience in this complex surgical technique [18].

11.3 Role of Chemotherapy in Localized Disease

Despite the fact that surgery represents the mainstay of the treatment of localized RPS [4, 19], compared to soft tissue sarcomas arising in other anatomic sites, RPS are characterized by a higher recurrence (50% at 5 years) and mortality rate (50% at 5 years) [20–24]. As of today, the extended surgical approach improved the curative rate compared to simple excision, but still a high proportion of patients will relapse and eventually die because of their sarcoma [4]. Thus, perioperative medical approaches remain appealing to reduce the rate of both local and distant recurrences. As mentioned, the risk of local failure and distant metastases are strictly related to the histology of RPS [21]. WDLPS are characterized by a relatively low local recurrence rate, negligible metastatic potential and favorable survival outcomes (even though WDLPS may locally recur years after the primary resection). On the contrary, intermediate-grade DDLPS display a tendency to recur locally and a low metastatic potential. High-grade DDLPS have a high risk of both local recurrence and distant metastases. LMS are characterized by an intermediate-to-high malignant potential with a significant risk of distant metastases, but meaningful and durable local control with adequate surgery. As a consequence, a perioperative approach in RPS should be tailored to histology. Clearly, chemotherapy needs to be considered in aggressive histologies, in order to reduce the risk of distant metastases. For example, DDLPS and LMS are likely the optimal histologies to be considered for perioperative chemotherapy.

The use of adjuvant chemotherapy in STS has been tested in several controlled trials with contrasting results, probably as a consequence of the heterogeneity of study populations. A first meta-analysis on adjuvant doxorubicin-based chemotherapy in localized STS of all sites showed a 10% improvement in recurrence-free survival, without a benefit in OS [25]. Later, in 2008 a meta-analysis including additional randomized clinical trials showed an improvement even in overall survival (HR 0.56) [26]. Thus, after acknowledging that these meta-analyses were mostly based on limb sarcomas, there are data to suggest in selected cases a role for an adjuvant treatment in RPS. In this regard, a very useful tool might be the above-mentioned nomogram to strengthen risk assessment. Secondly, histology is another key factor to support or weaken the role of an adjuvant therapy.

More recently, preliminary data of an international randomized clinical trial of histotype-tailored chemotherapy versus standard chemotherapy on high-risk STS of the extremities and trunk demonstrated an OS benefit for patients treated with three cycles of epirubicin and ifosfamide in the neoadjuvant setting [27]. This trial was closed before including all the planned patients, as an interim analysis showed a significant benefit in the standard chemotherapy arm. The design of the study compared three cycles of epirubicin (120 mg/m^2) and ifosfamide (9 g/m^2) with histology-driven chemotherapy regimens, in five STS histotypes (LMS, UPS, LPS, MPNST, and synovial sarcoma), given in the preoperative setting. This trial clearly shows that patients treated with anthracycline and ifosfamide have a statistically significant disease-free survival (62% vs. 38%) and OS benefit (89% vs. 64%) compared to the other arm. As a consequence of this study, the last European Society for Medical Oncology (ESMO) guidelines include the possibility of administering neoadjuvant chemotherapy with anthracycline and ifosfamide in patients with high grade STS of the trunk and extremity [4]. How these results may be applied to RPS is a matter of debate as is whether these data can be considered valid also for the adjuvant setting. Indeed, the study population was different for anatomical sites, and one of the commonest histotypes, DDLPS, was not included in the study. In principle, it seems reasonable to assume that if chemotherapy improves high-grade STS of the extremity, this could be applicable for sarcomas arising in other sites, on condition that high-risk tumors be selected. A prospective randomized trial would be greatly helpful in this context. Therefore, the EORTC Soft Tissue and Bone Sarcoma Group is planning a randomized study of neoadjuvant chemotherapy in RPS focusing on LMS and DDLPS. Few dedicated trials addressed the role of chemotherapy in the perioperative setting and most of these experiences are retrospective. In general several limitations affect these papers. In particular, these works tend to pool together different settings (first and relapsed presentations) and the use of chemotherapy has undoubtedly changed over the last 20 years even though doxorubicin is still the most active drug. Therefore, the trials are inconclusive on the role of chemotherapy and no definitive conclusions can be drawn. In a large retrospective nation-wide database, Jashodeep et al. could not show any impact of an adjuvant treatment after surgery. The authors acknowledge several limitations and emphasize that there might be a subgroup benefitting from chemotherapy after surgery [28]. A neoadjuvant experience was published by Gronchi et al. on 83 patients treated with ifosfamide 14 g/m^2 + radiotherapy (DFT 50.4 Gy) in the neoadjuvant setting. Patients were treated with three chemotherapy cycles followed by surgery at an interval of 4–6 weeks. Despite the fact the treatment was overall feasible, this trial does not allow definitive conclusions to be drawn due to the lack of a comparative group showing an OS of 63% at a median follow up of 7.5 year. Moreover, the use of radiotherapy makes any conclusion unsound [29].

11.4 Systemic Chemotherapy in Metastatic Settings

Metastatic disease in RPS requires an accurate evaluation by the multidisciplinary sarcoma board in order to define the goal of the treatment (neoadjuvant, palliative or curative) and to analyze every available instrument, including systemic and global therapy.

Despite the reported poor outcome for metastatic RPS, with a median OS of 16 months, the possibility of long-term survival and consequently of cure is still an opportunity to pursue [30]. Metastatic RPS includes two different clinical presentations both requiring upfront chemotherapy: systemic disease, with lung, liver and bone involvement and multifocal intra-abdominal disease, called abdominal sarcomatosis.

Systemic chemotherapy is the preferred first-line approach in both synchronous metastatic disease and in metachronous metastases, when they are not suitable for complete resection or appearing after a short disease-free interval. The chemotherapy regimen has to be defined on the basis of the treatment goal, evaluating the potential benefit and toxicity. A combination regimen can be offered in order to achieve surgical resectability, as this is associated to a higher response rate. A palliative chemotherapy regimen, usually based on a single agent, might be the best option in case of unresectable disease for disseminated pulmonary, hepatic or peritoneal metastases. In this section, we will concentrate on the pure palliative setting providing information based on histotypes and summarizing recent drug approvals and indications in STS as well as in RPS.

As reported in the Introduction, the first-line systemic treatment in palliative setting is represented by the single agent doxorubicin, alone or in combination with olaratumab. Indeed, this combination may well become the standard of care if the results of the phase III trial ANNOUNCE confirm the significant advantage in OS reported in the phase I/II trial (11.8 months) [13]. ESMO has already published an e-update concerning the new ESMO-MCBS (Magnitude of Clinical Benefit Scale) grading for olaratumab in unresectable or metastatic STS. Since the EORTC 62012 phase III trial did not show benefit in terms of OS by adding ifosfamide to doxorubicin, this combination remains a valid option whenever tumor shrinkage could be effective to relieve acute symptoms or preserve adjacent critical structures [4, 7]. There are, however, clinical presentations in which it may be desirable to achieve a greater tumor shrinkage as in symptomatic cases or when surgical complete resection may still be an option. In these situations and after tumor board discussion a combination between anthracycline and ifosfamide can be taken into account [7].

The best sequence to choose for second-, third- and further-line therapy is not defined, as for extremity STS. Histological subtype, tumor grading along with comorbidities, performance status and patient's preference represent the principal drivers to guide the decision-making process, in which patient expectancy and quality of life are crucial. In rare diseases, sharing the information and the available data with the patient and the family represents the cornerstone of the treatment choice. In some histotypes, for example WDLPS, characterized by indolent behavior or limited disease, an active surveillance can represent a correct policy, despite the fact that this proposal can be challenging to share with some patients.

The alkylating agent ifosfamide represents a valid second-line option, especially in LPS and MPNST. There is retrospective evidence suggesting that ifosfamide may be less active in LMS in which the use is increasingly less supported [10]. In recurrent RPS, previously treated with radical surgery, renal impairment can be an issue and can be an obstacle to this regimen [31]. Efficacy is related to the dose and modality of infusion, although in metastatic patients continuous infusion has better tolerance and manageability. Another hypothetical histotype is synovial sarcoma, a very chemosensitive histology where ifosfamide represents a reasonable option.

Three non-randomized phase II studies showed the efficacy of trabectedin in heavily pretreated patients, suggesting slightly more efficacy in LPS and LMS compared to other STS subtypes. [32–34] The randomized phase III trial comparing two different trabectedin regimens confirmed the advantage of the 24-hour infusion every 3 weeks with an increase in time to progression greater than 33% as compared to the previous chemotherapy in both LMS and LPS [35]. The study, which led to trabectedin approval by the FDA in 2015, showed 45% of risk reduction in disease progression or death compared to dacarbazine in LMS and LPS. Notwithstanding this result, dacarbazine remains an option for patients with LMS and SFT, where an association with doxorubicin may represent the first line of chemotherapy also in the advanced setting. As single agent, dacarbazine demonstrated a 17% response rate, associated with a very high level of tolerability and manageability.

Gemcitabine is used either alone or in combination with docetaxel. Since toxicity is considerably different, the use of the combination in the advanced setting should be thoroughly discussed according to the clinical context. The combination with docetaxel was explored in two randomized studies, the SARC study in STS and the French Sarcoma Group study in LMS [36, 37]. The results were conflicting and the real benefit of using the combination is still not defined, even in LMS. On the contrary, as a single agent, gemcitabine is extremely manageable and deserves great consideration in a nearly palliative setting as in advanced RPS. The schedule can be personalized and is particularly active in LMS and UPS.

Pazopanib, a multitarget tyrosine kinase inhibitor, is for the treatment of patients with advanced pretreated non-adipocytic sarcoma, demonstrating a statistically significant improvement in PFS compared to placebo without OS benefit (12.5 months with pazopanib vs. 10.7 months with placebo) [4, 11]. In 2016, eribulin, a marine-derived compound, was approved by the FDA and the EMA for the treatment of pretreated LPS. Eribulin showed a statistically significant improvement in OS over dacarbazine in the LPS cohort (15.6 months vs. 8.4 months) without differences in median PFS [38].

Currently, the median OS and PFS in metastatic RPS has been improving as a result of more aggressive approaches by the multidisciplinary sarcoma board and the multiple therapeutic choices. Overall, these results are likely due to several reasons. Clinicians have more further-line therapies which, although only marginally efficacious, may impact OS. However, it is the multidisciplinary approach that may yield the greatest advantage. Indeed, beyond optimal surgery and medical therapy a wise use of local treatments such as RITA and/or radiotherapy have always to be considered in an integrated clinical management. Only this complete knowledge of the pathological, clinical and therapeutic aspects of these diseases supports experts in reaching improved outcomes while respecting the quality of life of sarcoma patients.

References

1. Fletcher CDM, Bridge JA, Hogendoorn PCW, Mertens F (eds) (2013) WHO classification of tumours of soft tissue and bone. IARC Press, Lyon
2. Woll PJ, Reichardt P, Le Cesne A et al; EORTC Soft Tissue and Bone Sarcoma Group and the NCIC Clinical Trials Group Sarcoma Disease Site Committee (2012) Adjuvant chemotherapy with doxorubicin, ifosfamide, and lenograstim for resected soft-tissue sarcoma (EORTC 62931): a multicentre randomised controlled trial. Lancet Oncol 13(10):1045–1054

3. Toulmonde M, Bonvalot S, Méeus P et al; French Sarcoma Group (2014) Retroperitoneal sarcomas: patterns of care at diagnosis, prognostic factors and focus on main histological subtypes: a multicenter analysis of the French Sarcoma Group. Ann Oncol 25(3):735–742

4. Casali PG, Abecassis N, Bauer S et al (2018) Soft tissue and visceral sarcomas: ESMO-EURACAN Clinical Practice Guidelines for diagnosis, treatment and follow-up. Ann Oncol [Epub ahead of print] doi:10.1093/annonc/mdy096

5. van Houdt WJ, Zaidi S, Messiou C et al (2017) Treatment of retroperitoneal sarcoma: current standards and new developments. Curr Opin Oncol 29(4):260–267

6. Wagner AJ, Malinowska-Kolodziej I, Morgan JA et al (2010) Clinical activity of mTOR inhibition with sirolimus in malignant perivascular epithelioid cell tumors: targeting the pathogenic activation of mTORC1 in tumors. J Clin Oncol 28(5):835–840

7. Judson I, Verweij J, Gelderblom et al; European Organisation and Treatment of Cancer Soft Tissue and Bone Sarcoma Group (2014) Doxorubicin alone versus intensified doxorubicin plus ifosfamide for first-line treatment of advanced or metastatic soft-tissue sarcoma: a randomised controlled phase 3 trial. Lancet Oncol 15(4):415–423

8. Seddon B, Strauss SJ, Whelan J et al (2017) Gemcitabine and docetaxel versus doxorubicin as first-line treatment in previously untreated advanced unresectable or metastatic soft-tissue sarcomas (GeDDiS): a randomised controlled phase 3 trial. Lancet Oncol 18(10):1397–1410

9. Eriksson M (2010) Histology-driven chemotherapy of soft-tissue sarcoma. Ann Oncol 21(Suppl 7):vii270–vii276

10. Sleijfer S, Ouali M, van Glabbeke M et al (2010) Prognostic and predictive factors for outcome to first-line ifosfamide-containing chemotherapy for adult patients with advanced soft tissue sarcomas: an exploratory, retrospective analysis on large series from the European Organization for Research and Treatment of Cancer-Soft Tissue and Bone Sarcoma Group (EORTC-STBSG). Eur J Cancer 46(1):72–83

11. van der Graaf WT, Blay JY, Chawla SP et al; EORTC Soft Tissue and Bone Sarcoma Group; PALETTE study group (2012) Pazopanib for metastatic soft-tissue sarcoma (PALETTE): a randomised, double-blind, placebo-controlled phase 3 trial. Lancet 379(9829):1879–1886

12. Demetri GD, Schöffski P, Grignani G et al (2017) Activity of eribulin in patients with advanced liposarcoma demonstrated in a subgroup analysis from a randomized phase III study of eribulin versus dacarbazine. J Clin Oncol 35(30):3433–3439

13. Tap WD, Jones RL, Van Tine BA et al (2016) Olaratumab and doxorubicin versus doxorubicin alone for treatment of soft-tissue sarcoma: an open-label phase 1b and randomised phase 2 trial. Lancet 388(10043):488–497

14. Raut CP, Miceli R, Strauss DC et al (2016) External validation of a multi-institutional retroperitoneal sarcoma nomogram. Cancer 122(9):1417–1424

15. Trans-Atlantic RPS Working Group (2016) Management of recurrent retroperitoneal sarcoma (RPS) in the adult: a consensus approach from the Trans-Atlantic RPS Working Group. Ann Surg Oncol 23(11):3531–3540

16. Miura JT, Charlson J, Gamblin TC et al (2015) Impact of chemotherapy on survival in surgically resected retroperitoneal sarcoma. Eur J Surg Oncol 41(10):1386–1392

17. Tan MCB, Brennan MF, Kuk D et al (2016) Histology-based classification predicts pattern of recurrence and improves risk stratification in primary retroperitoneal sarcoma. Ann Surg 263(3):593–600

18. Bonvalot S, Cavalcanti A, Le Péchoux C et al (2005) Randomized trial of cytoreduction followed by intraperitoneal chemotherapy versus cytoreduction alone in patients with peritoneal sarcomatosis. Eur J Surg Oncol 31(8):917–923

19. Trans-Atlantic RPS Working Group (2015) Management of primary retroperitoneal sarcoma (RPS) in the adult: a consensus approach from the Trans-Atlantic RPS Working Group. Ann Surg Oncol 22(1):256–263

20. Gronchi A, Bonvalot S, Le Cesne A, Casali PG (2009). Resection of uninvolved adjacent organs can be part of surgery for retroperitoneal soft tissue sarcoma. J Clin Oncol 27(12):2106–2107

21. Gronchi A, Strauss DC, Miceli R et al (2016) Variability in patterns of recurrence after resection of primary retroperitoneal sarcoma (RPS): a report on 1007 patients from the multi-institutional collaborative RPS working group. Ann Surg 263(5):1002–1009

22. Gronchi A, Colombo C, Raut CP (2014) Surgical management of localized soft tissue tumors. Cancer 120(17):2638–2648

23. Pasquali S, Vohra R, Tsimopoulou I et al (2015) Outcomes following extended surgery for retroperitoneal sarcomas: results from a UK referral centre. Ann Surg Oncol 22(11): 3550–3556

24. Gronchi A, Miceli R, Shurell E et al (2013) Outcome prediction in primary resected retroperitoneal soft tissue sarcoma: histology-specific overall survival and disease free-survival nomogram built on major sarcoma center data sets. J Clin Oncol 31(13):1649–1655

25. Sarcoma Meta-analysis Collaboration (1997) Adjuvant chemotherapy for localised resectable soft-tissue sarcoma of adults: meta-analysis of individual data. Lancet 350 (9092):1647–1654

26. Pervaiz N, Colterjohn N, Farrokhyar F et al (2008) A systematic meta-analysis of randomized controlled trials of adjuvant chemotherapy for localized resectable soft-tissue sarcoma. Cancer 113(3):573–581

27. Gronchi A, Ferrari S, Quagliuolo V et al (2017) Histotype-tailored neoadjuvant chemotherapy versus standard chemotherapy in patients with high-risk soft-tissue sarcomas (ISG-STS 1001): an international, open-label, randomised, controlled, phase 3, multicentre trial. Lancet Oncol 18(6):812–822

28. Datta J, Ecker BL, Neuwirth MG et al (2017) Contemporary reappraisal of the efficacy of adjuvant chemotherapy in resected retroperitoneal sarcoma: evidence from a nationwide clinical oncology database and review of the literature. Surg Oncol 26(2):117–124

29. Gronchi A, De Paoli A, Dani C et al (2014) Preoperative chemo-radiation therapy for localised retroperitoneal sarcoma: a phase I-II study from the Italian Sarcoma Group. Eur J Cancer 50(4):784–792

30. Blay JY, van Glabbeke M, Verweij J et al (2003) Advanced soft-tissue sarcoma: a disease that is potentially curable for a subset of patients treated with chemotherapy. Eur J Cancer 39(1):64–69

31. Kim DB, Gray R, Li Z et al (2018) Effect of nephrectomy for retroperitoneal sarcoma on post-operative renal function. J Surg Oncol 117(3):425–429

32. Garcia-Carbonero R, Supko JG, Manola J et al (2004) Phase II and pharmacokinetic study of ecteinascidin 743 in patients with progressive sarcomas of soft tissues refractory to chemotherapy. J Clin Oncol 22(8):1480–1490

33. Le Cesne A, Blay JY, Judson I et al (2005) Phase II study of ET-743 in advanced soft tissue sarcomas: A European Organisation for the Research and Treatment of Cancer (EORTC) soft tissue and bone sarcoma group trial. J Clin Oncol 23(3):576–584

34. Yovine A, Riofrio M, Blay JY et al (2004) Phase II study of ecteinascidin-743 in advanced pretreated soft tissue sarcoma patients. J Clin Oncol 22(5):890–899

35. Demetri GD, Chawla SP, von Mehren M et al (2009) Efficacy and safety of trabectedin in patients with advanced or metastatic liposarcoma or leiomyosarcoma after failure of prior anthracyclines and ifosfamide: results of a randomized phase II study of two different schedules. J Clin Oncol 27(25):4188–4196

36. Maki RG, Wathen JK, Patel SR et al (2007) Randomized phase II study of gemcitabine and docetaxel compared with gemcitabine alone in patients with metastatic soft tissue sarcomas: results of Sarcoma Alliance for Research Through Collaboration study 002 [corrected]. J Clin Oncol 25(19):2755–2763

37. Pautier P, Floquet A, Penel N et al (2012) Randomized multicenter and stratified phase II study of gemcitabine alone versus gemcitabine and docetaxel in patients with metastatic or relapsed leiomyosarcomas: a Fédération Nationale des Centres de Lutte Contre le Cancer (FNCLCC) French Sarcoma Group Study (TAXOGEM study). Oncologist 17(9):1213–1220

38. Schöffski P, Chawla S, Maki RG et al (2016) Eribulin versus dacarbazine in previously treated patients with advanced liposarcoma or leiomyosarcoma: a randomised, open-label, multicentre, phase 3 trial. Lancet 387(10028):1629–1637

Predicting the Risk of Recurrence in Retroperitoneal Sarcoma

12

Dario Callegaro, Alessandro Gronchi, Andrea Napolitano, and Bruno Vincenzi

12.1 Introduction

12.1.1 The Biology of Recurrence in Retroperitoneal Sarcoma

Overall, soft tissue sarcomas comprise more than 60 different histologies, but five of them represent more than 90% of the retroperitoneal sarcoma (RPS):

- well-differentiated liposarcoma (WDLPS);
- dedifferentiated liposarcoma (DDLPS);
- leiomyosarcoma (LMS);
- solitary fibrous tumor (SFT);
- malignant peripheral nerve sheath tumor (MPNST).

These histologies are characterized by different biological behaviors with different early and late risks of local and distant recurrence [4].

Liposarcomas of the retroperitoneum are the most frequent histology, comprising more than 50% of RPS. DDLPS represent about 35% of all RPS. They can be intermediate- or high-grade tumors. The first group has a high tendency to local relapse (about 40% at 7 years), but low risk of distant metastases (about 10% for the same period). High-grade DDLPS, on the contrary, have the same 40% risk of local relapse at 7 years, but a significantly higher risk of distant metastases (DM) as well (about 30% at 5 years). For this reason, the 7-year overall survival of high-grade DDLPS is as low as 30%, compared to about 50% for intermediate-grade DDLPS [4]. WDLPS represent about 25% of all RPS [4]. They are low-grade tumors that commonly reach large dimensions before

D. Callegaro (✉)
Sarcoma Service, Department of Surgery, Fondazione IRCCS Istituto Nazionale dei Tumori
Milan, Italy
e-mail: dario.callegaro@istitutotumori.mi.it

V. Quagliuolo, A. Gronchi (Eds), *Current Treatment of Retroperitoneal Sarcomas*,
Updates in Surgery
DOI: 10.1007/978-88-470-3980-3_12, © Springer-Verlag Italia 2019

becoming symptomatic and so diagnosed. Survival for patients with WDLPS is about 80% at 7 years. Because of their relatively indolent nature, they have a limited early local recurrence (LR) potential but require long-term follow-up as they can recur locally decades after primary resection. At 7 years, LR can be as high as 30% [4].

Leiomyosarcomas represent about 20% of RPS. Most often they arise from major abdominal veins, in particular from the inferior vena cava, the renal veins and the gonadal veins. LMS are characterized by a high risk of DM and a low risk of local relapse. Indeed, about 50% of LMS patients develop metastatic lesions within the first 5 years, while only 10% will recur locally in the same timeframe. In this histology, the hematogenous spread more than the local status informs prognosis [4].

Solitary fibrous tumors represent about 6% of all RPS [4]. In the "classic" variant they are generally cured with adequate surgical resection. Nevertheless, about 10% of them present an aggressive behavior and harbor a metastatic potential (the so-called "malignant SFT"). The LR rate of retroperitoneal SFT is low compared to other histologies (about 10% at 7 years), and the survival at the same time point is around 80% [4].

Retroperitoneal MPNST represent about 3% of all RPS. They are characterized by a significant risk of both local relapse and DM and can occur in patients with neurofibromatosis [4].

Looking at these data, it is clear that the evaluation of the risk of relapse should take into account, among other factors, the specific histologic subtype of RPS, as the biology behind the different variants is substantially different.

12.2   From Individual Data to Individualized Prediction

12.2.1   Statistical End-points and Approaches for Predicting the Risk of Recurrence

The most commonly used end-point of recurrence is disease-free survival (DFS), also known as recurrence-free survival. DFS is defined as the interval between definitive treatment (surgery in the case of RPS) and local relapse, distant metastasis, or death, whichever occurs first. As site of relapse is often of particular interest, complementary end-points to DFS are also local relapse-free survival and metastases-free survival or the crude cumulative incidence of LR or DM. Overall survival (OS) — the interval between the date of definitive treatment and the date of death from any cause — and disease-specific mortality are often calculated to facilitate the interpretation of data and extrapolate how much relapse affects mortality.

Multivariate survival analysis can be divided into two broad categories: accelerated failure time models and proportional hazard approaches (including the semi-parametric Cox model and fully parametric approaches) [6].

Accelerated failure time models assume that the effect of a covariate is to accelerate or decelerate the survival curve by some constant [6]. This is especially appealing in a context where the final event analyzed is the result of a process with a known sequence of intermediary stages. Proportional hazard approaches on the other hand assume that the effect of a covariate is to multiply the hazard of an event by some constant, which implies that the relative risk in one subgroup compared to a baseline subgroup is constant over time. One of these models, the Cox proportional hazard model, is the most commonly used multivariate approach for analyzing survival time data in medical research [7].

The Cox model is reliable when the principal assumption of proportionality of hazards is tenable, and there is no concern for competing events, i.e. events whose occurrence preclude the occurrence of the primary event of interest [8]. When the outcome of interest, for example local or distant tumor relapse, is possibly unobserved due to the occurrence of a competing event, such as patient's death before developing a relapse, other models, such as the Fine and Gray model, should be preferred [9].

12.2.2 Tools for Recurrence Prediction: Nomograms

Nomograms were developed as graphical calculating devices that allow the analogic computation of a mathematical function. In biomedical research, especially in oncology, they can be used to translate the hazard ratio derived from survival analyses into a readily usable interface to predict the individualized risk of developing an event [10].

Traditionally, nomograms have a graduated scale for each covariate. The value of each covariate corresponds to a particular score, usually calculated drafting a straight line to another axis (the "point axis"). The sum of all the scores reflects the combined contribution of the covariates, which is converted into the outcome of interest. The inaccuracy intrinsically related to the use of the graphical instruments is nowadays overcome by the use of digital calculators that may be offered as a smartphone and/or tablet app or as a website.

The first step in developing a nomogram is the identification of a clear, focused and addressable question that needs a mathematical model to be answered. The selection of the variables (covariates) is the next important step, as exclusion of fundamental variables, as well as inclusion of unnecessary ones, can significantly affect the statistical model and the derived nomogram. Once derived, the nomogram needs to be validated in an unbiased setting to estimate its performance in terms of discriminative ability (i.e. capability to predict whether an individual will or will not develop the studied event or, among two individuals, who will develop the event first) and calibration (i.e. how close its predictions are to the observed outcome), as well as its applicability to discrete and diverse populations. Validation should ideally be performed on external datasets. Internal validation using cross-validation and bootstrapping – whereby the model is iteratively applied to randomly selected sample sets of the original cohort – remove some but not all the bias [10].

12.3   Nomograms for RPS Patients

The first nomogram to predict the 12-year sarcoma-specific death in patients affected by soft tissue sarcoma at all sites was developed in 2002 at the Memorial Sloan Kettering Cancer Center of New York [11]. The variables considered in this nomogram were age at diagnosis, tumor size, histologic grade, histologic subtype, depth, and site. From a statistical perspective, the nomogram was generated with a multivariable Cox regression model stratified on the "grade" variable, as this variable violated the proportional hazards assumption (i.e. had an effect that changed over time). Following this seminal work, several nomograms have been proposed to predict the outcome in soft tissue sarcoma patients, often in selected histologies, for example desmoid fibromatosis [13], liposarcoma [13], or synovial sarcoma [14, 15].

The first nomogram specific for RPS patients treated with surgery and curative intent was developed in 2010 by Anaya et al. [16]. Variables included in the nomogram were age (65 years cut-off), tumor size (15 cm cut-off), multifocality, completeness of resection, histology and tumor presentation (primary vs. recurrent). The predicted outcomes were median, 3- and 5-year OS. A multivariate Cox model was used to derive the nomogram. Although a turning point in predicting outcome in RPS patients, some limitations were present in this nomogram: first, 30% of the patients in the developing set had recurrent tumors, whose biological and histological differences compared to primary tumors could significantly confound the model, although the variable "tumor presentation" was used to capture this heterogeneity; second, the histological classification (WDLPS, DDLPS, other) limited the role of grade as a potential variable in the nomogram [16]. Moreover, age and tumor size were declined as categorical variables with specified cut-off values.

In the same year, Ardoino et al. developed a nomogram based on five covariates (age, grade, histology, tumor size, and margins) to predict 5- and 10-year OS in RPS patients [17]. In contrast to Anaya's model, in this model only patients with primary RPS were included, and age and size were managed as continuous variables. Interestingly, the relative hazard associated with tumor size increased up to 25 cm and decreased thereafter, probably reflecting the fact that larger tumors are typically WDLPS or intermediate-grade DDLPS, which have better prognosis compared to LMS or high-grade DDLPS. Extending the interval observation to 10 years allowed better capturing of the late recurrences of selected histotypes, such as WDLPS. Weaknesses of this model are the confinement of WDLPS and DDLPS within the same "liposarcomas" group and the relatively small size of the patients' cohort.

Importantly, neither the Anaya nor the Ardoino nomograms have been externally validated, and they only predict OS, lacking specific tumor-related predictions, such as the probability of LR, DM, or DFS.

Most of these limitations were overcome in 2013, when Gronchi et al. published the results of an international multicentric collaborative effort that led to the development and validation of two nomograms specific for primary RPS patients to predict 7-year OS and 7-year DFS (Fig. 12.1) [18]. For these nomograms, the development cohort comprised more than 500 patients from three major sarcoma centers, mitigating some selection bias likely present in single institutional series. Importantly, these patients received the most current treatment strategies, such as aggressive frontline surgery. On the other hand, due to the limited patient follow-up, predictions were limited to 7 years. These OS and DFS nomograms were based on multivariable Cox regression models. Covariates of the OS nomogram included grade, tumor size, histology, patient age, multifocality, and extent of surgical resection. The same variables except for extent of surgical resection and patient age were used in the DFS nomogram. Patient age and tumor size were modelled as continuous variables, and histological subtypes were expanded to seven different categories according to the latest WHO classification system [18].

Importantly, these models underwent three independent external validations maintaining a good discriminative ability [18–20] and have been included in the latest edition of the American Joint Committee on Cancer/Union for International Cancer Control classification of RPS. Finally, both nomograms have also been integrated into an app for smartphone, "Sarculator", allowing clinicians the opportunity to have real time access to this predictive tool (Fig. 12.2).

In 2016, Tan et al. developed novel RPS-specific nomograms to predict disease specific death, LR and DM probability at 3, 5, and 10 years after surgery [21]. The major strengths of these nomograms are the extensive long-term follow-up in data collection and the existence of separate predictors of LR and DM. On the other hand, the development series came from a single institution where the standard of RPS care has been represented by surgical resection limited to overtly infiltrated organs usually without adjuvant therapies and has not changed over the years. Therefore, in the absence of any external validations, the applicability of these nomograms outside the developing institution remains only hypothetical. Moreover, the two-tiered grading system used in these models does not allow discerning the outcome of intermediate-grade vs. high-grade tumors.

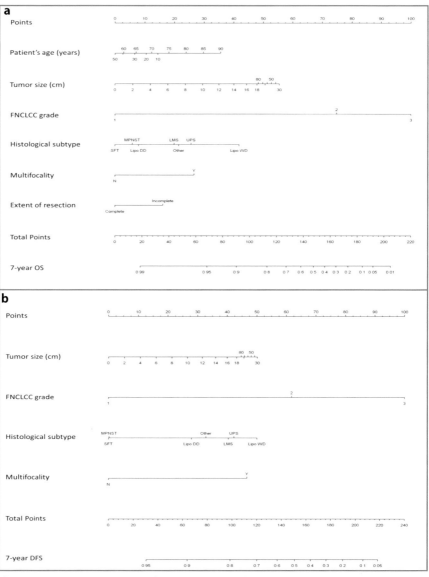

Fig. 12.1 These nomograms allow for the calculation of the 7-year probability of overall survival (**a**) and disease-free survival (**b**) after surgical resection of a primary retroperitoneal sarcoma.

To use OS nomogram, locate the patient's age on the corresponding axis and draw a line straight up to the "points" axis to determine the score associated with that age. Repeat this process for all the other covariates (tumor size, FNCLCC grade, histological subtype, multifocality, extent of resection). Sum the score of each covariate and find the total score on the "total points" axis. Draw a line straight down to the 7-year OS axis to obtain the probability.

OS, overall survival; *DFS*, disease-free survival; *SFT*, solitary fibrous tumor; *MPNST*, malignant peripheral nerve sheath tumor; *Lipo DD*, dedifferentiated liposarcoma; *LMS*, leiomyosarcoma; *UPS*, undifferentiated pleomorphic sarcoma; *Lipo WD*, well-differentiated liposarcoma; *FNCLCC*, Fédération Nationale des Centres de Lutte Contre le Cancer. Reprinted with permission from [18].

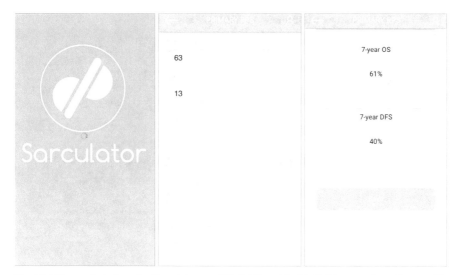

Fig. 12.2 Screenshots from the Sarculator app (Digital Forest S.r.l.). In this example, a 63-year-old patient operated on for a 13-cm G2 leiomyosarcoma (no multifocality, complete resection) has a predicted 7-year overall survival of 61% and a predicted 7-year disease-free survival of 40%. The Sarculator app is available for free download from the official stores

A comparative analysis of available RPS nomograms is detailed in Table 12.1 [22].

12.4   Conclusions

In summary, recent efforts have led to the creation of several predictive tools for RPS patients. For patients with primary RPS, nomograms from Gronchi et al. (Fig. 12.1) are currently the most robust and the only validated tools. In selected cases and with caution, Anaya's nomogram may provide some prognostic information for patients with recurrent RPS and Tan's nomograms might inform on the risk of DM or LR.

In the future, nomograms specifically dedicated to unresectable, metastatic or recurrent patients, or which could be used in the preoperative setting are clearly needed. During the 2018 Connective Tissue Oncology Society meeting, new prognostic nomograms specific for recurrent RPS were presented by the Trans-Atlantic Retroperitoneal Sarcoma Working Group (TARPSWG, www.tarpswg.org) and will likely become available soon. Moreover, the integration of genomic, radiomic and immunological variables, such as the CINSARC molecular signature [24], is likely to improve the performance of prognostic nomograms in the future. Finally, the individualized risk prediction offered

Table 12.1 Nomograms for retroperitoneal sarcoma patients

Study	Patient population		Development series characteristics		
Authors (year)	**N. of patients**	**Median FU**	**Selection criteria**	**Time frame**	**N. of centers**
Anaya et al. (2010) [16]	343 *of which:* – pre/postop CT 155 (45%) – pre/postop RT 111 (32%) – incomplete resection 35 (10%)	50 months	Primary or recurrent, non-metastatic, resected	1996– 2006	1
Ardoino et al. (2010) [17]	192 *of which:* – pre/postop CT 57 (29.6%) – pre/postop RT 58 (30.2%) – incomplete resection 14 (7.3%)	55 months	Primary, localized, resected	1985– 2007	1
Gronchi et al. (2013) [18]	523 *of which:* – pre/postop CT 207 (39.6%) – pre/postop RT 193 (36.9%) – incomplete resection 48 (9.2%) 475	45 months	Primary, localized, resected	1999– 2009	3
Tan et al. (2016) [21]	632 *of which:* – pre/postop CT 121 (18%)* – pre/postop RT 54 (8%)* – incomplete resection 58 (9%)* 574 632	40 months*	Primary, localized, resected	1982– 2010	1

pre/postop CT, preoperative/postoperative chemotherapy; *pre/postop RT*, preoperative/postoperative radiotherapy; *FU*, follow-up; *OS*, overall survival; *WDLPS*, well-differentiated liposarcoma; *DDLPS*, dedifferentiated-liposarcoma; *FNCLCC*, Fédération Nationale des Centres de Lutte Contre le Cancer

Nomograms details			Internal validation	External validation
Predicted outcomes	**Covariates**	**Multivariable model**	**Concordance index**	**Concordance index**
Median, 3- and 5-year OS	histology (WDLPS, DDLPS, other), completeness of resection, age (dichotomic, cutoff at 65 years), multifocality, tumor size (dichotomic, cutoff at 15 cm), presentation (primary vs recurrent)	Cox	0.73 (0.71–0.75)[#]	n/a
5- and 10-year OS	histology (5 categories), FNCLCC grade, size (continuous), margins (complete vs incomplete), age (continuous)	Piecewise exponential	0.73	n/a
7-year OS	FNCLCC grade, tumor size (continuous), histology (7 categories), patient's age (continuous), multifocality (y vs n), extent of resection (complete vs incomplete)	Cox	0.74	0.67–0.73[#]
7-year DFS	FNCLCC grade, tumor size (continuous), histology (7 categories), multifocality (y vs n)	Cox	0.71	0.68–0.69[#]
3-, 5- and 10-year DSD	histology (7 categories), extent of resection (R0/R1 vs R2), number of organs resected (dichotomic, cutoff at 3 organs), size (3 categories), RT (y vs n)	Fine and Gray	0.71 (0.66–0.74)[#]	n/a
3-, 5- and 10-year LR rate	histology (7 categories), size (3 categories), age (dichotomic, cutoff at 65 years), resection (R0 vs R1), location (pelvis vs other), vascular resection (y vs n), number of resected organs (dichotomic, cutoff at 3 organs).	Fine and Gray	0.71 (0.67–0.75)[#]	n/a
3-, 5- and 10-year DR rate	histology (7 categories), number of resected organs (0 vs 1-2 vs 3 organs), size (3 categories), RT (y vs n), vascular resection (y vs n).	Fine and Gray	0.74 (0.69–0.77)[#]	n/a

(France); *DFS*, disease-free survival; *LR*, local recurrence; *DR*, distant recurrence; *n/a*, not available
* Data referring to the overall cohort of 675 patients; [#] 95% confidence interval

Adapted with permission from [22]

by nomograms may well become a new criterion to select RPS patients in randomized clinical trials.

References

1. Lewis JJ, Leung D, Casper ES et al (1999) Multifactorial analysis of long-term follow-up (more than 5 years) of primary extremity sarcoma. Arch Surg 134(2):190–194
2. Morrison BA (2003) Soft tissue sarcomas of the extremities. Proc (Bayl Univ Med Cent) 16(3):285–290
3. Bonvalot S, Raut CP, Pollock RE et al (2012) Technical considerations in surgery for retroperitoneal sarcomas: position paper from E-Surge, a master class in sarcoma surgery, and EORTC-STBSG. Ann Surg Oncol 19(9):2981–2991
4. Gronchi A, Strauss DC, Miceli R et al (2016) Variability in patterns of recurrence after resection of primary retroperitoneal sarcoma (RPS): a report on 1007 patients from the Multi-institutional Collaborative RPS Working Group. Ann Surg 263(5):1002–1009
5. MacNeill AJ, Miceli R, Strauss DC et al (2017) Post-relapse outcomes after primary extended resection of retroperitoneal sarcoma: a report from the Trans-Atlantic RPS Working Group. Cancer 123(11):1971–1978
6. Bradburn MJ, Clark TG, Love SB, Altman DG (2003) Survival analysis part II: multivariate data analysis – an introduction to concepts and methods. Br J Cancer 89(3):431–436
7. Cox DR (1972) Regression models and life tables. J R Stat Soc Series B Stat Methodol 34(2):187–220
8. Dignam JJ, Zhang Q, Kocherginsky M (2012) The use and interpretation of competing risks regression models. Clin Cancer Res 18(8):2301–2308
9. Fine JP, Gray RJ (1999) A proportional hazards model for the subdistribution of a competing risk. J Am Stat Assoc 94(446):496–509
10. Balachandran VP, Gonen M, Smith JJ, DeMatteo RP (2015) Nomograms in oncology: more than meets the eye. Lancet Oncol 16(4):e173–e180
11. Kattan MW, Leung DH, Brennan MF (2002) Postoperative nomogram for 12-year sarcoma-specific death. J Clin Oncol 20(3):791–796
12. Crago AM, Denton B, Salas S et al (2013) A prognostic nomogram for prediction of recurrence in desmoid fibromatosis. Ann Surg 258(2):347–353
13. Dalal KM, Kattan MW, Antonescu CR et al (2006) Subtype specific prognostic nomogram for patients with primary liposarcoma of the retroperitoneum, extremity, or trunk. Ann Surg 244(3):381–391
14. Canter RJ, Qin LX, Maki RG et al (2008) A synovial sarcoma-specific preoperative nomogram supports a survival benefit to ifosfamide-based chemotherapy and improves risk stratification for patients. Clin Cancer Res 14(24):8191–8197
15. Callegaro D, Miceli R, Mariani L et al (2017) Soft tissue sarcoma nomograms and their incorporation into practice. Cancer 123(15):2802–2820
16. Anaya DA, Lahat G, Wang X et al (2010) Postoperative nomogram for survival of patients with retroperitoneal sarcoma treated with curative intent. Ann Oncol 21(2):397–402
17. Ardoino I, Miceli R, Berselli M et al (2010) Histology-specific nomogram for primary retroperitoneal soft tissue sarcoma. Cancer 116(10):2429–2436
18. Gronchi A, Miceli R, Shurell E et al (2013) Outcome prediction in primary resected retroperitoneal soft tissue sarcoma: histology-specific overall survival and disease-free survival nomograms built on major sarcoma center data sets. J Clin Oncol 31(13):1649–1655
19. Raut CP, Miceli R, Strauss DC et al (2016) External validation of a multi-institutional retroperitoneal sarcoma nomogram. Cancer 122(9):1417–1424

20. Chou YS, Liu CY, Chang YH et al (2016) Prognostic factors of primary resected retro-peritoneal soft tissue sarcoma: analysis from a single Asian tertiary center and external validation of Gronchi's nomogram. J Surg Oncol 113(4):355–360

21. Tan MC, Brennan MF, Kuk D et al (2016) Histology-based classification predicts pattern of recurrence and improves risk stratification in primary retroperitoneal sarcoma. Ann Surg 263(3):593–600

22. Callegaro D, Miceli R, Gladdy RA (2018) Prognostic models for RPS patients – Attempting to predict patient outcomes. J Surg Oncol 117(1):69–78

23. Chibon F, Lagarde P, Salas S et al (2010) Validated prediction of clinical outcome in sarcomas and multiple types of cancer on the basis of a gene expression signature related to genome complexity. Nat Med 16(7):781–787

Multimodal Management of Metastatic Disease

13

Alexia F. Bertuzzi, Umberto Cariboni, Matteo M. Cimino, and Guido Torzilli

13.1   Introduction

Despite complete initial resection, more than 50% of patients treated for a retroperitoneal sarcoma (RPS) will relapse and about 20–25% will develop distant metastases. In the presence of resectable local recurrence surgery should be the first choice, representing a concrete chance of complete surgical remission and, in some selected cases, of cure. However, a successful complete resection is a difficult goal to achieve given the risk of further relapses and we will have a significant proportion of patients with unresectable or borderline resectable abdominal disease or metastatic disease. The latter includes a systemic disease characterized either by lung/liver involvement or by a multifocal intra-abdominal diffusion, so called sarcomatosis. Despite multimodal management, the outcome for metastatic RPS remains poor with a median overall survival (OS) of 16 months and a reported 5-year OS around 5% [1]. The appropriate treatment strategy for every patient with unresectable or metastatic RPS should be the result of a global consensus by a multidisciplinary sarcoma tumor board with expertise in the available surgical and medical options taking into account aspects related to the rarity and the heterogeneity of this disease (histotype, grading, interval free, extension), to the patient (age, performance status, comorbidities) and to the final goal of the treatment.

First of all, a correct disease and patient assessment has to be conducted. A pathological review of the primary tumor represents the first step, including the diagnosis made by a sarcoma center given the frequent variability between

A.F. Bertuzzi (✉)
Department of Medical Oncology and Hematology, Humanitas Clinical and Research Center
Rozzano, Milan, Italy
e-mail: alexia.bertuzzi@cancercenter.humanitas.it

V. Quagliuolo, A. Gronchi (Eds), *Current Treatment of Retroperitoneal Sarcomas*,
Updates in Surgery
DOI: 10.1007/978-88-470-3980-3_13, © Springer-Verlag Italia 2019

institutions [2]. Because often the patient has received a previous treatment, the sarcoma board needs to review the surgical details of the resection, the chemotherapy regimen and the cumulative dose of drugs administered (e.g., anthracyclines and ifosfamide) as well as the dose and the field of radiotherapy.

The actual stage of the disease has to be defined by appropriate imaging, often driven by the histological type [3]. An abdominal/pelvic computed tomography (CT) scan is the preferred imaging modality in order to evaluate the intra-abdominal peritoneal disease. Abdomen magnetic resonance imaging (MRI) may be indicated to clarify the presence of recurrence rather than post-treatment fibrosis/scarring or to address some neurovascular involvement especially in paravertebral lesions. Liver MRI may also be indicated in the definition of liver metastases supported by a triphasic CT scan or plain liver ultrasound. The role of fluorine-18 fluorodeoxyglucose positron emission tomography (^{18}F-FDG-PET) is still debated in sarcoma but surely it can help to identify peritoneal disease or, in some histological subtype, it can clarify the presence of bone involvement. In cases of a first diagnosis of advanced RPS, a biopsy needs to be performed. Usually the biopsy of an intra-abdominal mass should be done under CT guidance, without transgressing the peritoneal cavity and by an expert radiologist. Hepatic or pulmonary lesions require a histological diagnosis in few cases only, where the imaging is unclear or when the disease-free interval is very long.

Patient assessment requires a deep knowledge of comorbidities, performance status, presence of sequelae from previous surgical or medical treatments (e.g., cardiac or renal impairment), disability, and symptoms of the current status of the disease. The patient's role is extremely important in the multidisciplinary management of rare diseases and represents an essential part of the decision-making process. Extensive information regarding the treatment goal and the balance between benefit and cost of the therapy characterizes the approach to sarcoma patients, especially in an advanced setting.

The multidisciplinary sarcoma team has to be composed by a medical, surgical, radiation oncologist specialist, by a sarcoma pathologist and an expert radiologist. The sarcoma board should take into account all the information provided regarding the disease and the patient as reported above. A tailored patient strategy is recommended, sharing with the patient preferences and goals of care.

Cases of locally advanced or synchronous oligometastatic disease (potentially resectable) represent the best setting, in which a favorable response to a 'neoadjuvant' treatment could make the patient eligible for resection of the primary tumor and/or metastasectomy, which represents the only possibility for long-term survival in metastatic RPS.

In order to carry out the surgical resection, 'neoadjuvant' chemotherapy alone or combined with radiation should always be considered, although no randomized trials have been reported. First-line chemotherapy or an observation period without treatment in some selected histotypes should also be considered in order to understand the tumor biology and evaluate the appropriateness of an aggressive local treatment.

Polychemotherapy should be the first choice because the response rate (RR) could really impact the chances of cure, by downsizing the primary tumor and guaranteeing radical surgery. This effect can be observed especially in some chemosensitive histotypes such as synovial sarcoma or leiomyosarcoma.

A patient undergoing metastasectomy should meet at least two fundamental criteria: complete resection of the primary tumor and all metastatic sites either completely resectable or controllable with local therapies [4]. Currently, other less invasive local therapies – such as radiofrequency ablation and stereotactic body radiotherapy – are considered acceptable alternatives, with fewer complications and shorter systemic treatment interruption [5, 6]. The selection of patients candidate to this approach requires the presence of some favorable prognostic features such as low volume disease, a disease-free interval of 12 months or longer and a confirmed response to or prolonged stable disease on systemic therapy.

Conversely, patients with multimetastatic disease and/or an abdominal sarcomatosis (unresectable) should be directed to a pure palliative setting, including systemic chemotherapy in cases of good performance status or only best supportive care [7]. The goal of our choice should be prolongation of an acceptable quality of life, balancing the potential benefits of systemic treatment against expected toxicity. Sequential single-drug chemotherapy will probably be less toxic without significantly impairing survival. The combined treatment should be considered even in a palliative setting if the tumor shrinkage could be effective to relieve acute symptoms (painful bulky abdominal mass or intestinal subocclusion) or to preserve adjacent critical structures [8].

Network treatment guidelines recommend anthracycline-based chemotherapy – primarily with doxorubicin – as first-line treatment (RR around 16–27% and a median OS of 7.3 to 12.7 months) [9].

Interestingly, the most recent studies in metastatic soft tissue sarcoma showed an improvement in progression-free survival and OS compared with the previous published trials, suggesting that clinical expertise favor a better selection of drugs and a more aggressive approach with less dose reduction or delays. Furthermore, a competent multidisciplinary approach even in the palliative setting can include local therapies such radiotherapy or surgery, associated with longer OS [10].

Focusing on histotype and tailored regimens, we can give some general indications to be considered in expert hands and in the setting of palliative chemotherapy. Well-differentiated liposarcoma (WDLPS) and dedifferentiated liposarcoma (DDLPS), the most common liposarcoma subtypes, are considered relatively chemotherapy-resistant, with 12% of objective RR with an anthracycline-based regimen and a median OS of 15 months [11]. A higher sensitivity to chemotherapy is reported for myxoid liposarcoma (48%) compared to DDLPS (25%) [12]. Ifosfamide represents a good second-line choice with RR from 23% to 32% for DDLPS, even in pretreated patients [13]. The RR for continuous-infusion ifosfamide is 19% versus 45% for the daily bolus schedule, and seems particularly active in synovial sarcoma [14].

Trabectedin, approved by the European Commission for the treatment of soft tissue sarcomas in 2007 and by the Food and Drug Administration (FDA) in 2015 in patients with unresectable or metastatic liposarcoma (LPS) and leiomyosarcoma (LMS), showed a statistically significant 45% reduction in the risk of disease progression or death with respect to dacarbazine. Consistent with the good tolerance profile, the therapeutic benefit of continued disease control is one of the most important strengths of trabectedin, supporting its use even beyond six cycles [15, 16].

The FDA and the European Medicines Agency (EMA) have recently approved eribulin for the treatment of pretreated LPS. Eribulin showed a statistically significant improvement in OS over dacarbazine in the LPS cohort (15.6 months versus 8.4 months). There was no difference in median progression-free survival [17].

In LMS, the second most common subtype developing in the retroperitoneum, associated with a high metastatic potential, doxorubicin plus dacarbazine represents a valid option, based on the retrospective European Organisation for Research and Treatment of Cancer (EORTC) evidence showing no convincing activity of ifosfamide in either this histotype or in solitary fibrous tumor [18–20]. In the initial studies, the combination of doxorubicin and dacarbazine was noted to have a clinical RR of 41%, reduced to 16–30% in the most recent randomized trials [21, 22]. The combination of gemcitabine and docetaxel had 53% objective response and an advantage versus the single agent gemcitabine [23–25]. The GeDDiS trial found no indication of a superior response to gemcitabine and docetaxel in either LMS or uterine LMS with respect to the other histotypes and confirmed no difference between this combination and doxorubicin as first-line treatment [26].

Finally, pazopanib, a multitargeted tyrosine kinase inhibitor, has been approved by the US FDA in April 2012 for the treatment of patients with advanced pretreated non-adipocytic sarcoma, showing a statistically significant improvement in progression-free survival (HR=0.35) without overall survival benefit [27].

13.2   Hepatic Resection for Liver Metastases

Hepatic resection for liver metastases from colorectal and neuroendocrine cancers is widely accepted in the multimodal approach of these solid tumors and associated with a better prognosis [28, 29]. The benefit in non-colorectal and non-neuroendocrine liver metastases (NCNNLM) is still debated and the outcome depends on the histology of the primary lesion. The NCNNLM definition dates back to 1995 and includes mainly metastases from gastric and breast cancer and melanoma [30]. Only few retrospective series on RPS metastases were published since the late 90s, limited by small patient numbers, inclusion of patients with different histologies and short median follow-up.

Unlike extremity and trunk soft tissue sarcomas, liver metastases from primary visceral and RPS are common, from 20% to 60% [31] and chemotherapy or chemoembolization are not very effective. A recent paper analyzed the ten largest studies conducted on NCNNLM, in which the postoperative mortality and morbidity rates were reported to be 05% and 1833%, respectively [32].

With regard to metastatic sarcoma, the largest study reported 3- and 5-year OS rates of 50–65% and 13–46%, respectively, with a median OS of 24–72 months; the median number of lesions ranged from 1 to 3. The rate of major resections (>3 adjacent segments) ranged from 25% to 61%. Negative risk factors for OS in this cohort were a time of <24 months from the diagnosis of the primary tumor to the time of liver metastases, non-gastrointestinal stromal tumor (non-GIST) histology, LMS histology, extrahepatic disease, and positive resection margins (Table 13.1).

Lang et al. reported one of the largest series of 26 LMS patients receiving a total of 34 liver resections for hepatic metastases from 1982 to 1996. Gastrointestinal stromal tumor (GIST) might be included because it was considered LMS before 1993. No details were given about the specific outcome of these patients but there were 23 first, 9 second, and 2 third liver resections [33]. The retrospective analysis published by De Matteo et al. showed similar survival after hepatic resection in GIST or intestinal LMS compared to other sarcoma histologies. The only positive prognostic factor at multivariate analysis was a disease-free interval (DFI) greater than two years [34]. In 2006, Pawlik et al. reported on 66 cases of hepatic resection for sarcoma with 22 (33%) patients with RPS or abdominal sarcoma as the primary lesion treated with surgery and/or radiofrequency ablation (RFA). At multivariate analysis, patients treated with surgery alone showed an improved OS compared to patients treated with RFA only or RFA plus surgery (median OS 54 vs. 32 months). Patients treated with chemotherapy showed a better outcome [35]. Marudanayagam et al. reported on a series of 36 patients treated with hepatic resection for sarcomas, only two of them with liver metastases from RPS. The positive prognostic factors were non-LMS histology, negative margins and low-intermediate grade at histology [36].

In conclusion, we can state that hepatic resection for sarcoma must be chosen on a case-by-case basis after a multidisciplinary team discussion. A long DFI and response to chemotherapy are the principal criteria for referring patients for hepatic resection. R0 resection and the clearance of incidental extrahepatic disease must always be attempted to guarantee an improved OS and DFI.

Table 13.1 Summary of studies of patients treated with surgery for liver metastases from sarcomas

Author	Year	Period	N. of patients	Lesions (median n.)	MH	Median OS (months)	3-year OS	5-year OS	Factors associated with worse OS
Lang et al. [33]	2000	1982–1996	26	2	30	32 (R0 resection), 21 (R1/2 resection)	NR	13	NR
De Matteo et al. [34]	2001	1982–2000	56	1	25	39	50	30	Time to liver metastasis from the primary tumor diagnosis ≤24 months
Pawlik et al. [35]	2006	1996–2005	53	3	41	47	65	27	Non-GIST
Marudanayagam et al. [36]	2011	1997–2009	36	1	61	26	48	32	Leiomyosarcoma

MH, major hepatectomy; *OS*, overall survival; *NR*, not reported; *Non-GIST*, non-gastrointestinal stromal tumor.

Repeated hepatectomy can be performed in selected patients due to low rate of response to chemotherapy.

13.3 Pulmonary Resection for Lung Metastases

Pulmonary metastases develop in 20% of patients with a diagnosis of soft tissue sarcoma and 40% in bone sarcoma. Due to low chemotherapy RR, the application of only systemic treatment options is limited in clinical practice. Therefore, surgical resection of isolated pulmonary metastases is considered standard treatment and is related to an improvement in life expectancy [37, 38]. Pulmonary metastasectomy has to be defined by a sarcoma board team, which also decides if it is appropriate to combine chemotherapy to the surgery (as neoadjuvant, adjuvant or both). The decision is based on many parameters as well as the DFI, the number of metastases, growth rate, and histology.

Many studies have confirmed some common characteristics influencing the prognosis in the case of lung resections, such as age, comorbidities, aggressiveness of tumor recurrence, histology of the primary sarcoma, DFI, size and number of lung lesions, unilateral disease, complete resection of metastases, intrathoracic location of metastases and responsiveness to chemotherapy. On the other hand, negative prognostic factors were represented by male gender, bilateral disease, high French Federation of Cancer Centers (FNCLCC) grading (calculated on differentiation, mitotic count and tumor necrosis), and high-risk histologies [39].

Many publications have demonstrated how DFI represents one of the most important prognostic factors: a DFI greater than 12 months is associated with a substantial increase of OS in contrast with a DFI lower than 12 months [40]. Another prognostic factor is the number of lung lesions [41]. Interestingly, there is not yet a specific score able to establish the correlation between lesion number and OS: some studies reported less than four metastases, others less than three and some only one (5-year survival was 70% for one, 46% for two to three, and 22% for more than three) [6]. Other important predictors are complete surgical resection, size of the nodes (<3 cm or >3 cm) and negative surgical margins (the 5-year survival for those with negative resection margins was 82%), which decrease the risk of disease dissemination [40–43]. Histology is relevant: lung metastases from a bone sarcoma have a better prognosis compared to metastases from a soft tissue sarcoma [44].

The studies report that the patients receiving an adjuvant, or a neoadjuvant chemotherapy or radiotherapy have worse OS compared to patients who have only had surgery. This conclusion could be due to the bias that these treatments are offered to patients with negative prognostic factors, such as size >3 cm, multiple and/or deep localization or bilateral disease.

There are different surgical approaches to the pulmonary metastasectomy, including video-assisted thoracic surgery (VATS) or open thoracotomy. Multiple studies confirm the potential advantage of the VATS approach. On the other hand, for those patients who have multiple nodes, located deeply or with other negative parameters an open approach is indicated, which improves the possibility to achieve an R0 resection thanks to bimanual palpation and resection of occult metastases [39, 42, 44, 45].

References

1. Blay J-Y, van Glabbeke M, Verweij J et al (2003) Advanced soft-tissue sarcoma: a disease that is potentially curable for a subset of patients treated with chemotherapy. Eur J Cancer 39(1):64–69
2. Trans-Atlantic Retroperitoneal Sarcoma Working Group (TARPSWG) (2018) Management of metastatic retroperitoneal sarcoma: a consensus approach from the Trans-Atlantic Retroperitoneal Sarcoma Working Group (TARPSWG). Ann Oncol 29(4):857–871
3. Messiou C, Moskovic E, Vanel D et al (2017) Primary retroperitoneal soft tissue sarcoma: imaging appearances, pitfalls and diagnostic algorithm. Eur J Surg Oncol 43(7):1191–1198
4. Abdalla EK, Pisters PW (2002) Metastasectomy for limited metastases from soft tissue sarcoma. Curr Treat Options Oncol 3(6):497–505
5. Navarria P, Ascolese AM, Cozzi L et al (2015) Stereotactic body radiation therapy for lung metastases from soft tissue sarcoma. Eur J Cancer 51(5):668–674
6. Jones RL, McCall J, Adam A et al (2010) Radiofrequency ablation is a feasible therapeutic option in the multi modality management of sarcoma. Eur J Surg Oncol 36(5):477–482
7. Anaya DA, Lahat G, Liu J et al (2009) Multifocality in retroperitoneal sarcoma: a prognostic factor critical to surgical decision-making. Ann Surg 249(1):137–142
8. Judson I, Verweij J, Gelderblom H et al; European Organisation and Treatment of Cancer Soft Tissue and Bone Sarcoma Group (2014) Doxorubicin alone versus intensified doxorubicin plus ifosfamide for first-line treatment of advanced or metastatic soft-tissue sarcoma: a randomised controlled phase 3 trial. Lancet Oncol 15(4):415–423
9. Bramwell V, Anderson D, Charette M; Sarcoma Disease Site Group (2003) Doxorubicin-based chemotherapy for the palliative treatment of adult patients with locally advanced or metastatic soft tissue sarcoma. Cochrane Database Syst Rev (3):CD003293
10. Falk AT, Moureau-Zabotto L, Ouali M et al; Groupe Sarcome Français-Groupe d'Etude des Tumeurs Osseuses (2015) Effect on survival of local ablative treatment of metastases from sarcomas: a study of the French sarcoma group. Clin Oncol (R Coll Radiol) 27(1):48–55
11. Italiano A, Toulmonde M, Cioffi A (2012) Advanced well-differentiated/dedifferentiated liposarcomas: role of chemotherapy and survival. Ann Oncol 23(6):1601–1607
12. Jones RL, Fisher C, Al-Muderis O, Judson IR (2005) Differential sensitivity of liposarcoma subtypes to chemotherapy. Eur J Cancer 41(18):2583–2860
13. Sanfilippo R, Bertulli R, Marrari A et al (2014) High-dose continuous-infusion ifosfamide in advanced well-differentiated/dedifferentiated liposarcoma. Clin Sarcoma Res 4(1):16
14. Patel SR, Vadhan-Raj S, Papadopolous N et al (1997) High-dose ifosfamide in bone and soft tissue sarcomas: results of phase II and pilot studies – dose-response and schedule dependence. J Clin Oncol 15(6):2378–2384
15. Demetri GD, von Mehren M, Jones RL et al (2016) Efficacy and safety of trabectedin or dacarbazine for metastatic liposarcoma or leiomyosarcoma after failure of conventional chemotherapy: results of a phase III randomized multicenter clinical trial. J Clin Oncol 34(8):786–793

16. Le Cesne A, Blay J-Y, Domont J et al (2015) Interruption versus continuation of trabectedin in patients with soft-tissue sarcoma (T-DIS): a randomised phase 2 trial. Lancet Oncol 16(3):312–319

17. Schöffski P, Chawla S, Maki RG et al (2016) Eribulin versus dacarbazine in previously treated patients with advanced liposarcoma or leiomyosarcoma: a randomised, open-label, multicentre, phase 3 trial. Lancet 387(10028):1629–1637

18. Gottlieb JA, Benjamin RS, Baker LH et al (1976) Role of DTIC (NSC-45388) in the chemotherapy of sarcomas. Cancer Treat Rep 60(2):199–203

19. Sleijfer S, Ouali M, van Glabbeke M et al (2010) Prognostic and predictive factors for outcome to first-line ifosfamide-containing chemotherapy for adult patients with advanced soft tissue sarcomas: an exploratory, retrospective analysis on large series from the European Organization for Research and Treatment of Cancer Soft-Tissue and Bone Sarcoma Group (EORTC-STBSG). Eur J Cancer 46(1):72–83

20. Casali PG, Abecassis N, Bauer S et al (2018) Soft tissue and visceral sarcomas: ESMO-EURACAN Clinical Practice Guidelines for diagnosis, treatment and follow-up. Ann Oncol [Epub ahead of print] doi:10.1093/annonc/mdy096

21. Gottlieb JA, Baker LH, Quagliana JM et al (1972) Chemotherapy of sarcomas with a combination of adriamycin and dimethyl triazeno imidazole carboxamide. Cancer 30(6):1632–1638

22. Antman K, Crowley J, Balcerzak SP et al (1993) An intergroup phase III randomized study of doxorubicin and dacarbazine with or without ifosfamide and mesna in advanced soft tissue and bone sarcomas. J Clin Oncol 11(7):1276–1285

23. Maki RG, Wathen JK, Patel SR et al (2007) Randomized phase II study of gemcitabine and docetaxel compared with gemcitabine alone in patients with metastatic soft tissue sarcomas: results of Sarcoma Alliance for Research Through Collaboration study 002 [corrected]. J Clin Oncol 25(19):2755–2763

24. Hensley ML, Maki R, Venkatraman E et al (2002) Gemcitabine and docetaxel in patients with unresectable leiomyosarcoma: results of a phase II trial. J Clin Oncol 20(12):2824–2831

25. Pautier P, Floquet A, Penel N et al (2012) Randomized multicenter and stratified phase II study of gemcitabine alone versus gemcitabine and docetaxel in patients with metastatic or relapsed leiomyosarcomas: a Fédération Nationale des Centres de Lutte Contre le Cancer (FNCLCC) French Sarcoma Group Study (TAXOGEM study). Oncologist 17(9):1213–1220

26. Seddon B, Strauss SJ, Whelan J et al (2017) Gemcitabine and docetaxel versus doxorubicin as first-line treatment in previously untreated advanced unresectable or metastatic soft-tissue sarcoma (GeDDiS): a randomised controlled phase 3 trial. Lancet Oncol 18(10):1397–1410

27. van der Graaf WT, Blay JY, Chawla SP et al; EORTC Soft Tissue and Bone Sarcoma Group; PALETTE study group (2012) Pazopanib for metastatic soft-tissue sarcoma (PALETTE): a randomised, double-blind, placebo-controlled phase 3 trial. Lancet 379(9829):1879–1886

28. Touzios JG, Kiely JM, Pitt SC et al (2005) Neuroendocrine hepatic metastases: does aggressive management improve survival? Ann Surg 241(5):776–783; discussion 783–785

29. Choti MA, Sitzmann JV, Tiburi MF et al (2002) Trends in long-term survival following liver resection for hepatic colorectal metastases. Ann Surg 235(6):759–766

30. Schwartz SI (1995) Hepatic resection for noncolorectal nonneuroendocrine metastases. World J Surg 19(1):72–75

31. Mudan SS, Conlon KC, Woodruff JM et al (2000) Salvage surgery for patients with recurrent gastrointestinal sarcoma: prognostic factors to guide patient selection. Cancer 88(1):66–74

32. Takemura N, Saiura A (2017) Role of surgical resection for non-colorectal non-neuroendocrine liver metastases. World J Hepatol 9(5):242–251

33. Lang H, Nussbaum KT, Kaudel P et al (2000) Hepatic metastases from leiomyosarcoma: a single-center experience with 34 liver resections during a 15-year period. Ann Surg 231(4):500–505

34. DeMatteo RP, Shah A, Fong Y et al (2001) Results of hepatic resection for sarcoma metastatic to liver. Ann Surg 234(4):540–547
35. Pawlik TM, Vauthey JN, Abdalla EK et al (2006) Results of a single-center experience with resection and ablation for sarcoma metastatic to the liver. Arch Surg 141(6):537–543; discussion 543–544
36. Marudanayagam R, Sandhu B, Perera MT et al (2011) Liver resection for metastatic soft tissue sarcoma: an analysis of prognostic factors. Eur J Surg Oncol 37(1):87–92
37. Choong PF, Pritchard DJ, Rock MG et al (1995) Survival after pulmonary metastasectomy in soft tissue sarcoma. Prognostic factors in 214 patients. Acta Orthop Scand 66(6):561–568
38. Pastorino U, Buyse M, Friedel G et al; International Registry of Lung Metastases (1997) Long-term results of lung metastasectomy: prognostic analyses based on 5206 cases. J Thorac Cardiovasc Surg 113(1):37–49
39. Billingsley KG, Burt ME, Jara E et al (1999) Pulmonary metastases from soft tissue sarcoma: analysis of patterns of diseases and postmetastasis survival. Ann Surg 229(5):602–610; discussion 610–612
40. Roth JA, Putnam JB Jr, Wesley MN, Rosenberg SA (1985) Differing determinants of prognosis following resection of pulmonary metastases from osteogenic and soft tissue sarcoma patients. Cancer 55(6):1361–1366
41. Casson AG, Putnam JB, Natarajan G et al (1992) Five-year survival after pulmonary metastasectomy for adult soft tissue sarcoma. Cancer 69(3):662–668
42. Kim S, Ott HC, Wright CD et al (2011) Pulmonary resection of metastatic sarcoma: prognostic factors associated with improved outcomes. Ann Thorac Surg 92(5):1780–1786; discussion 1786–1787
43. Putnam JB Jr, Roth JA, Wesley MN et al (1984) Analysis of prognostic factors in patients undergoing resection of pulmonary metastases from soft-tissue sarcoma. J Thorac Cardiovasc Surg 87(2):260–268
44. Kon Z, Martin L (2011) Resection for thoracic metastases from sarcoma. Oncology (Williston Park) 25(12):1198–1204
45. García Franco CE, Torre W, Tamura A et al (2010) Long-term results after resection for bone sarcoma pulmonary metastases. Eur J Cardiothoracic Surg 37(5):1205–1208

Postoperative Surveillance in Retroperitoneal Sarcomas

14

Alessandro Comandone, Antonella Boglione, and Teresa Mele

14.1 The Meaning of Surveillance

In oncological patients, surveillance refers to the periodic radiological and clinical evaluations performed in radically resected patients, who are macroscopically disease free [1–5]. Postoperative surveillance procedures have the primary aim to decrease mortality and improve quality of life through early detection of local relapse or distant metastases. However, in most tumors (breast, colon, ovarian. non-small-cell lung cancer), the early detection of relapsing or metastatic disease before the onset of symptoms seldom improves the overall survival [1–5]. Another goal of follow-up measures in oncology is the diagnosis and management of late toxicities and morbidities related to neoadjuvant or adjuvant therapies (both radiotherapy and chemotherapy) [1–5]. Psychosocial support for patients and their families is the third aim of post-treatment surveillance [1–3].

In several common neoplasms (breast, colorectal cancers, prostate carcinoma) many follow-up guidelines have been issued to guide clinicians in surveillance. Unfortunately, such recommendations in soft tissue sarcomas (STS) are not universally accepted.

In breast cancer, for instance, the American Society of Clinical Oncology (ASCO) and the European Society for Medical Oncology (ESMO) recommend minimal follow-up procedures such as anamnesis, clinical examination, limited blood tests, serological markers and annual mammography [3–5]. Data from the literature and guidelines suggest that intensive follow-up measures – with abdominal computed tomography (CT), ultrasound (US), chest X-ray or

A. Comandone (✉)
Oncology Department, Humanitas Gradenigo Hospital
Turin, Italy
e-mail: alessandro.comandone@gradenigo.it

V. Quagliuolo, A. Gronchi (Eds), *Current Treatment of Retroperitoneal Sarcomas*, Updates in Surgery
DOI: 10.1007/978-88-470-3980-3_14, © Springer-Verlag Italia 2019

165

pulmonary CT, and bone scan – do not improve survival or quality of life [3–5]. The duration of follow-up is also an open question [3–5].

In STS of the extremities, clinical examination of the operated area, supported by US or magnetic resonance imaging (MRI) of the surrounding soft tissues and chest X-ray or CT scan of the lungs are generally accepted as common diagnostic tests during surveillance [6–12]. As the risk of recurrence is dependent on histology, grading and size of the tumor, follow-up measures are based on these characteristics [6–8, 10–12]. Radically resected low-grade sarcoma should be monitored every 6–12 months for at least 5 years; high-grade sarcomas need a stricter surveillance (every 3–4 months). Follow-up can be stopped or delayed after 3 years [6–12].

14.2 Retroperitoneal Sarcomas

In retroperitoneal sarcomas (RPS) medium survival after complete resection is 103 months as opposed to 18 months in patients who undergo an incomplete resection [1, 13]. Low-grade tumors allow for a longer survival: 149 months versus 33 months in high-grade sarcomas [1]. Volume of RPS is another independent prognostic factor: tumors with size <15 cm have a better prognosis than sarcomas >15 cm. Due to the aforementioned factors, local relapse is a common event (4–68% of cases) [1, 13, 14]. Lastly, second and/or further relapses have a poorer prognosis compared to primary tumors, even after resection. One should also consider that surgery on relapsing tumor rarely leads to complete resection. Many surgeons in referral centers agree that the first intervention is strategic for the cure of patients, and after relapse there is no hope for a definitive cure [1, 13–20]. Distant metastases are less common than in STS of the extremities: liver and lung metastases account for 15% of the cases. Few data are reported on the effect of metastasectomy on survival [21, 22]. No specific study addressing the question of the best follow-up protocol for RPS has yet been published. Most of the guideline recommendations come from mono-institutional, observational, non-randomized studies in which extremity sarcomas, RPS and visceral sarcomas – sometimes including gastrointestinal stromal tumors (GIST) – are considered [6–12].

The main characteristics to be considered in RPS are depicted in Tables 14.1 and 14.2 [1, 2, 13–16]. Clinicians have to discern surveillance following the first resection or after iterative surgery. In the latter case, since surgery cannot be curative, there is a high risk of further relapses [1, 2, 13–20]. Even after the first surgical intervention, despite "complete" resection, the 5- and 10-year survival rates are 51% and 36%, respectively, showing a high number of early and late relapses [13–20]. Local recurrences mostly occur within 2 years from

Table 14.1 Tumor characteristics in retroperitoneal soft tissue sarcomas

Characteristics	Epidemiology
Histology	
Liposarcomas	50%
Leiomyosarcomas	20–25%
MPNST	15%
Round cells/Undifferentiated	5%
Other	3%
Grade	
1	32%
2	34%
3	30%
Type of surgery	
R0	47%
R1	26%
R2	10%
Tumor size	
<15 cm	37%
>15 cm	63%
Metastasis at diagnosis	
No	85%
Yes	15%

MPNST, malignant peripheral nerve sheath tumor

Table 14.2 Patient characteristics to be considered in assessing the prognosis of retroperitoneal sarcomas

- Age (≤65 years, >65 years)
- Performance status
- Comorbidities
- Polypharmacy
- Previous interventions for retroperitoneal sarcoma and number of previous surgeries
- Previous treatments (surgery only; neoadjuvant chemotherapy or chemo + radiotherapy; adjuvant chemotherapy or chemo + radiotherapy)

the initial surgery [13–20]. When relapsed, repeated surgery rarely leads to a complete cure, but the surgical approach on local relapse is recommended, as it leads to a longer time to progression of the disease [13–16]. In non-resectable sarcomas, palliative chemotherapy can be offered. Median survival is 8 months for patients who received exclusive chemotherapy and >14 months for a palliative treatment, even without radical resection [23–25].

Clinical history and examination are the first actions to be taken in RPS surveillance [6, 7, 9–11]. The history can reveal abdominal discomfort, pain, bowel disturbance, but only occasionally these symptoms are useful for an early diagnosis of relapse [6, 7, 9]. The clinical examination rarely succeeds in detecting a small volume recurrence [6, 7, 9–11]. No blood test or serological markers are useful in the postoperative surveillance of RPS or of any type of sarcoma. These tumors do not secrete biochemical substances useful for early disease detection. Lactate dehydrogenase is sometimes claimed as a serological marker for STS, but it is extensively expressed in body tissues, such as blood cells and muscles. Also, it is not specific for RPS or STS in general [6, 7, 9–11].

Consequently, radiological follow up is mandatory in RPS [6–12]. Nevertheless, it is not easy to differentiate a small volume relapse from postoperative scarring or fibrosis in the surgical field [6–12, 26]. A US scan is not appropriate due to its low sensitivity, and surveillance must include a CT scan or MRI of the abdomen [6–12, 26]. There are no differences between the two examinations in the detection of local relapses [6–12, 26]. Conversely, lung metastases are a rare event (<15% of cases) and can be diagnosed by chest X-ray (preferred option in UK, Canadian and Dutch guidelines) [2, 6, 9, 10] or by CT scan with/without contrast enhancement [6, 7, 26]. We also have to take into account the radiation risk, particularly for younger patients, and the impact of the iodine-based contrast medium in patients who have undergone nephrectomy as a result of a multivisceral surgery. Multiple sequential CT scan examinations repeated for at least 5 years might cause concern, and the abdominal follow-up can be performed with MRI with gadolinium as contrast medium [9, 26]. Positron-emission tomography (PET) has been used in the attempt to detect small recurrences of RPS in the postoperative fibrotic scar. The sensitivity does not exceed 60% and the specificity is around 75% [6, 7, 9, 10, 27]. As a consequence, at the present time PET cannot be considered a routine tool to detect early relapse in RPS [27].

14.3   Timing of Follow-up in Retroperitoneal Sarcoma

Surveillance timing is pursued in order to plan visits and radiological imaging at regular intervals, according to the sarcoma's characteristics and the patient's condition [6, 7, 9–12].

In low-grade sarcomas (well-differentiated and dedifferentiated liposarcomas) the consensus among the experts suggests repeating the CT scan or MRI every 6 months for a minimum of 5 years. Chest X-ray as well as a pulmonary CT scan should be repeated every 6–12 months. Some experts recommend continuing with postoperative surveillance up to 10 years after the operation [6, 7, 9–12].

In the case of high-grade sarcomas (leiomyosarcoma, round cell sarcomas, undifferentiated sarcomas) CT or MRI should be done every 3–4 months for 2 years and then every 4–6 months for 3 years and every 12 months thereafter. Chest CT of the lungs with/without contrast enhancement must be repeated every 6 months. Moreover, such strict follow-up is also recommended in relapsed disease of any grade [6, 7, 9–12].

14.4   Results of the Follow-up

Relapsing or metastatic disease can be faced in several different ways. Local recurrence must be considered for resection. Many studies demonstrated that a high percentage of patients experience a prolonged time to progression when local relapses can be macroscopically resected [1, 2, 13–16, 18, 19]. Further recurrences have less chances of being successfully resected, and currently iterative surgery can be recommended in low-grade liposarcoma only [1, 2, 13, 15, 16]. In cases of metastatic dissemination of RPS, non-resectable lung metastases treated with chemo- or radiotherapy are associated with a median survival ranging from 6 to 12 months [16, 17, 21]. Conversely, if a complete resection is feasible, about 25% of patients are alive at 5 years [1, 2, 16, 17, 21]. On the other hand, one series of patients who underwent resection of hepatic metastases reported 100% of recurrence rate [22]. In cases of liver involvement, neither a surgical approach nor ablative techniques are currently advised in international guidelines [22]. Chemotherapy for unresectable disease has been extensively investigated. Polychemotherapy compared with monotherapy improves response rate and progression-free survival, but no differences in overall survival have been recorded [23–25].

14.5   Conclusions

According to the available evidence, postoperative surveillance in RPS is a common practice in oncology. The appropriate follow-up strategy includes medical history, physical examination, CT scan or MRI of the abdomen and X-ray or CT scan of the lungs [6, 7, 9–11]. Early detection of local recurrence as well as lung metastases can improve the percentage of complete resections and consequently overall survival. Quality of life is also increased in patients who are regularly followed up [6–11]. RPS surveillance strategies need to be evaluated in prospective trials. However, an accurate follow-up is currently recommended and prescribed in daily clinical practice.

References

1. Youssef E, Fontanesi J, Mott M et al (2002) Long-term outcome of combined modality therapy in retroperitoneal and deep-trunk soft-tissue sarcoma: analysis of prognostic factors. Int J Radiat Oncol Biol Phys 54(2):514–519
2. Windham TC, Pisters PW (2005) Retroperitoneal sarcomas. Cancer Control 12(1):36–43
3. Khatcheressian JL, Hurley P, Bantug E et al; American Society of Clinical Oncology (2012) Breast cancer follow-up and management after primary treatment: American Society of Clinical Oncology clinical practice guideline update. J Clin Oncol 31(7):961–965
4. Runowicz CD, Leach CR, Henry NL et al (2016) American Cancer Society/American Society of Clinical Oncology breast cancer survivorship care guideline. J Clin Oncol 34(6):611–635
5. Senkus E, Kyriakides S, Ohno S et al (2015) Primary breast cancer: ESMO clinical practice guidelines for diagnosis, treatment and follow-up. Ann Oncol 26(Suppl 5):v8–v30
6. Casali PG, Abecassis N, Bauer S et al (2018) Soft tissue and visceral sarcomas: ESMO-EURACAN Clinical Practice Guidelines for diagnosis, treatment and follow-up. Ann Oncol [Epub ahead of print] doi:10.1093/annonc/mdy096
7. National Comprehensive Cancer Network Guidelines. Soft tissue sarcoma. https://www.nccn.org
8. Messiou C, Moskovic E, Vanel D et al (2017) Primary retroperitoneal soft tissue sarcoma: imaging appearances, pitfalls and diagnostic algorithm. Eur J Surg Oncol 43(7):1191–1198
9. Grimer R, Judson I, Peake D, Seddon B (2010) Guidelines for the management of soft tissue sarcomas. Sarcoma 2010:506182
10. Alberta Health Services. Follow-up surveillance of soft tissue sarcoma. http://www.albertahealthservices.ca
11. Whooley BP, Mooney MM, Gibbs JF, Kraybill WG (1999) Effective follow-up strategies in soft tissue sarcoma. Semin Surg Oncol 17(1):83–87
12. Kane JM 3rd (2004) Surveillance strategies for patients following surgical resection of soft tissue sarcomas. Curr Opin Oncol 16(4):328–332
13. Gutierrez JC, Perez EA, Franceschi D et al (2007) Outcomes for soft-tissue sarcoma in 8249 cases from a large state cancer registry. J Surg Res 141(1):105–114
14. Gronchi A, Miceli R, Shurell E et al (2013) Outcome prediction in primary resected retroperitoneal soft tissue sarcoma: histology-specific overall survival and disease-free survival nomograms built on major sarcoma center data sets. J Clin Oncol 31(13):1649–1655
15. Porter GA, Baxter NN, Pisters PW (2006) Retroperitoneal sarcoma: a population-based analysis of epidemiology, surgery, and radiotherapy. Cancer 106(7):1610–1616
16. Catton CN, O'Sullivan B, Kotwall C et al (1994) Outcome and prognosis in retroperitoneal soft tissue sarcoma. Int J Radiat Oncol Biol Phys 29(5):1005–1010
17. Gronchi A, Strauss DC, Miceli R et al (2016) Variability in patterns of recurrence after resection of primary retroperitoneal sarcoma (RPS): a report on 1007 patients from the Multi-institutional Collaborative RPS Working Group. Ann Surg 263(5):1002–1009

18. Bonvalot S, Rivoire M, Castaing M et al (2009) Primary retroperitoneal sarcomas: a multivariate analysis of surgical factors associated with local control. J Clin Oncol 27(1):31–37
19. Lewis JJ, Leung D, Woodruff JM, Brennan MF (1998) Retroperitoneal soft-tissue sarcoma: analysis of 500 patients treated and followed at a single institution. Ann Surg 228(3): 355–365
20. Strauss DC, Hayes AJ, Thway K et al (2010) Surgical management of primary retroperitoneal sarcoma. Br J Surg 97(5):698–706
21. Saltzman DA, Snyder CL, Ferrell KL et al (1993) Aggressive metastasectomy for pulmonic sarcomatous metastases: a follow-up study. Am J Surg 166(5):543–547
22. Jaques DP, Coit DG, Casper ES, Brennan MF (1995) Hepatic metastases from soft-tissue sarcoma. Ann Surg 221(4):392–397
23. Toulmonde M, Bonvalot S, Ray-Coquard I, French Sarcoma Group (2014) Retroperitoneal sarcomas: patterns of care in advanced stages, prognostic factors and focus on main histological subtypes: a multicenter analysis of the French Sarcoma Group. Ann Oncol 25(3):730–734
24. Noujaim J, van Der Graaf WT, Jones RL (2015) Redefining the standard of care in metastatic leiomyosarcoma. Lancet Oncol 16(4):360–362
25. Judson J, Verweij J, Gelderblom H et al; European Organisation and Treatment of Cancer Soft Tissue and Bone Sarcoma Group (2014) Doxorubicin alone versus intensified doxorubicin plus ifosfamide for first-line treatment of advanced or metastatic soft-tissue sarcoma: a randomised controlled phase 3 trial. Lancet Oncol 15(4):415–423
26. Francis IR, Cohan RH, Varma DGK, Sondak VK (2005) Retroperitoneal sarcomas. Cancer Imaging 5(1):89–94
27. Messa C, Landoni C, Pozzato C, Fazio F (2000) Is there a role for FDG PET in the diagnosis of muscoloskeletal neoplasms? J Nucl Med 41(10):1702–1703

Towards a Global Collaboration: the Trans-Atlantic Retroperitoneal Sarcoma Working Group

15

Alessandro Gronchi and Vittorio Quagliuolo

15.1 Past and Present

The contemporary era for the management of retroperitoneal sarcoma starts at the end of the first decade of the 21st century, when two major sarcoma groups reported the outcome of primary retroperitoneal sarcoma patients treated by not only complete but wider resections, incorporating adherent organs and soft tissue even without evidence of gross invasion at the time of surgery. This concept of a "compartmental" or extended resection was similar to that used in extremity soft tissue sarcoma in which the overlying skin, subcutaneous fat and adherent muscle are taken to provide a margin of normal tissue surrounding the tumor. They showed a significant reduction of local recurrence [1, 2] and – in a later manuscript – a significant improvement of overall survival [3]. These reports generated intense debate among the major sarcoma centers in Europe and North America [4–11], subsequently addressed by follow-up data [3, 12].

During this time, in part from the debate on the extent of resection, members from the participating institutions began to join together to form what would soon be called the Trans-Atlantic Retroperitoneal Sarcoma Working Group (TARPSWG) [13]. In 2013, the group formally convened for the first time on the occasion of the European Society of Medical Oncology (ESMO) meeting to update the guidelines on sarcoma and gastrointestinal stromal tumor [14]. The common goal was to better understand and optimize the treatment of retroperitoneal sarcoma (RPS) through multi-institutional collaboration.

A. Gronchi (✉)
Sarcoma Service, Department of Surgery, Fondazione IRCCS Istituto Nazionale dei Tumori
Milan, Italy
e-mail: alessandro.gronchi@istitutotumori.mi.it

V. Quagliuolo, A. Gronchi (Eds), *Current Treatment of Retroperitoneal Sarcomas,*   173
Updates in Surgery
DOI: 10.1007/978-88-470-3980-3_15, © Springer-Verlag Italia 2019

The collaborative efforts of TARPSWG have in recent years provided several contributions which have changed the surgical approach to RPS. Technical considerations for surgery in RPS (e.g., extended resection) have been reported for the first time and hands-on, practical courses have been sponsored by the group to educate other surgeons [15]. Consensus management guidelines for primary, recurrent and metastatic RPS have also been reported [16–18]. Combining data from the TARPSWG member institutions, nomograms to predict patient outcome after resection were developed and validated, specifically for primary and recurrent RPS [19, 20]. These multi-institutional nomograms data are in fact now available on smartphones through a free, downloadable application called the "Sarculator" (http://www.sarculator. com/). In addition, the primary RPS nomogram is mentioned as the best tool to stage RPS patients in the 8th edition of the American Joint Committee on Cancer (AJCC) staging manual.

In 2016, data from eight TARPSWG institutions for 1007 patients with primary RPS were reported, currently the largest series to date [21]. The data from this study and other contemporary studies [22–24] highlighted the value of histologic subtype as an important predictor for pattern of recurrence (e.g., local vs. distant). As a consequence, histologic subtype is now considered in the initial strategy, including the extent of surgery.

Several other manuscripts followed, addressing postoperative morbidity and mortality of these complex and extended procedures in general [25] and with a focus on specific procedures, such as pancreaticoduodenectomy [26], or on post-recurrence outcomes [27].

Finally, this collaboration was one of the main drivers to the successful conclusion of the recruitment of the first randomized trial on this disease (see below).

15.2   Future Directions

Overall, despite recent improvements and changes in the approach to surgical management of RPS, these tumors still remain challenging to treat effectively. Further efforts are needed to improve patient outcomes in this rare disease.

Specifically, the role of radiation therapy for local control in RPS remains to be better defined. The next likely major historical landmark in the management

RPS will be the results of an ongoing randomized prospective multicenter trial (STRASS, NCT01344018) comparing neoadjuvant radiation therapy followed by resection versus resection alone in RPS patients. Accrual is now complete and preliminary results are expected by late-mid 2019. Subgroup analysis by histologic subtype will be especially helpful.

The role of systemic therapy will be the next "frontier" to address. Thanks to the unique collaboration, a randomized study on neoadjuvant chemotherapy in a subgroup of patients affected by RPS at high risk of distant spread is now under preparation to follow STRASS (the so called STRASS-2).

Further developments will require deeper understanding of disease biology in RPS through laboratory-based research.

For such a rare disease, multi-institutional collaboration is critical and continues through groups such as TARPSWG. Institutional membership in TARPSWG has grown almost three-fold since its inception and continues to increase, with inclusion of not only surgical but also medical and radiation oncologists and pathologists to essentially recapitulate the multidisciplinary team of physicians that are typically involved in the management of an RPS patient. A collective, prospective database has been maintained (RESAR) since January 2017, with more than 400 patients already included. A tissue repository is also planned.

In addition, TARPSWG will likely begin to go "beyond the Atlantic" to include sarcoma referral centers in other countries (e.g., Asia) as a truly global collaboration in RPS. Some Asian centers from South Korea and China, Taiwan, Singapore, India, as well as Australia and other countries have already expressed their interest in joining. A more formalized group across the present societies and different continents (Connective Tissue Oncology Society, Society of Surgical Oncology, European Society of Surgical Oncology, etc.) will likely have to be set up. However, its growth and possible formalization will have to preserve at any cost its friendly environment and mutual trust, which have been the main driver of its success (Fig. 15.1).

In conclusion, the evolution of surgical management in RPS has progressed from historical descriptions of cases at autopsy to complete resection with minimal operative mortality in the majority of patients at sarcoma referral centers. These large and often dramatic tumors nonetheless remain challenging to treat effectively; however, with integration of non surgical therapies, continued research and collaborative efforts for this rare disease, the future appears promising.

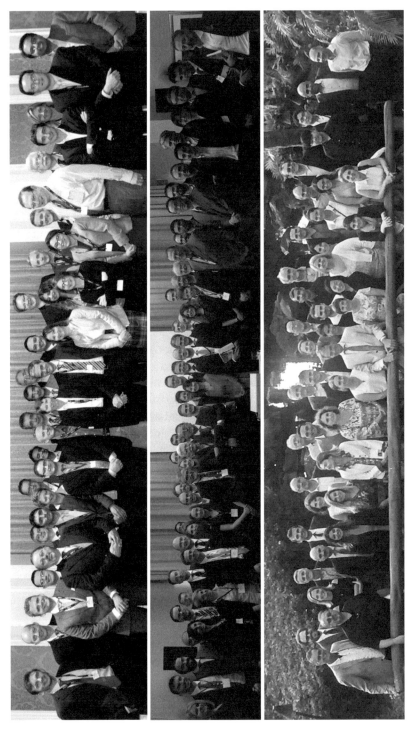

Fig. 15.1 The Trans-Atlantic Retroperitoneal Sarcoma Working Group (TARPSWG) at the annual meeting of the Connective Tissue Oncology Society in 2015 in Salt Lake City (*upper row*), in 2016 in Lisbon (*middle row*) and in 2017 in Maui (*lower row*)

References

1. Gronchi A, Lo Vullo S, Fiore M et al (2009) Aggressive surgical policies in a retrospectively reviewed single-institution case series of retroperitoneal soft tissue sarcoma patients. J Clin Oncol 27(1):24–30
2. Bonvalot S, Rivoire M, Castaing M et al (2009) Primary retroperitoneal sarcomas: a multivariate analysis of surgical factors associated with local control. J Clin Oncol 27(1):31–37
3. Gronchi A, Miceli R, Colombo C et al (2012) Frontline extended surgery is associated with improved survival in retroperitoneal low- to intermediate-grade soft tissue sarcomas. Ann Oncol 23(4):1067–1073
4. Pisters PW (2009) Resection of some – but not all – clinically uninvolved adjacent viscera as part of surgery for retroperitoneal soft tissue sarcomas. J Clin Oncol 27(1):6–8
5. Gronchi A, Bonvalot S, Le Cesne A, Casali PG (2009) Resection of uninvolved adjacent organs can be part of surgery for retroperitoneal soft tissue sarcoma. J Clin Oncol 27(12):2106–2107; author reply 2107–2108
6. Raut CP, Swallow CJ (2010) Are radical compartmental resections for retroperitoneal sarcomas justified? Ann Surg Oncol 17(6):1481–1484
7. Mussi C, Colombo P, Bertuzzi A et al (2011) Retroperitoneal sarcoma: is it time to change the surgical policy? Ann Surg Oncol 18(8):2136–2142
8. Gronchi A, Pollock RE (2011) Surgery in retroperitoneal soft tissue sarcoma: a call for a consensus between Europe and North America. Ann Surg Oncol 18(8):2107–2110
9. Gronchi A, Pollock RE (2013) Quality of local treatment or biology of the tumor: which are the trump cards for loco-regional control of retroperitoneal sarcoma? Ann Surg Oncol 20(7):2111–2113
10. Fairweather M, Wang J, Jo VY et al (2018) Surgical management of primary retroperitoneal sarcomas: rationale for selective organ resection. Ann Surg Oncol 25(1):98–106
11. Strauss DC, Renne SL, Gronchi A (2018) Adjacent, adherent, invaded: a spectrum of biologic aggressiveness rather than a rationale for selecting organ resection in surgery of primary retroperitoneal sarcomas. Ann Surg Oncol 25(1):13–16
12. Callegaro D, Miceli R, Brunelli C et al (2015) Long-term morbidity after multivisceral resection for retroperitoneal sarcoma. Br J Surg 102(9):1079–1087
13. Tseng WW, Pollock RE, Gronchi A (2016) The Trans-Atlantic Retroperitoneal Sarcoma Working Group (TARPSWG): "Red wine or white"? Ann Surg Oncol 23(13):4418–4420
14. ESMO/European Sarcoma Network Working Group (2014) Soft tissue and visceral sarcomas: ESMO clinical practice guidelines for diagnosis, treatment and follow-up. Ann Oncol 25:(Suppl 3):iii102–iii112
15. Bonvalot S, Raut CP, Pollock RE et al (2012) Technical considerations in surgery for retroperitoneal sarcomas: position paper from E-Surge, a master class in sarcoma surgery, and EORTC-STBSG. Ann Surg Oncol 19(9):2981–2991
16. Trans-Atlantic RPS Working Group (2015) Management of primary retroperitoneal sarcoma (RPS) in the adult: a consensus approach from the Trans-Atlantic RPS Working Group. Ann Surg Oncol 22(1):256–263
17. Trans-Atlantic RPS Working Group (2016) Management of recurrent retroperitoneal sarcoma (RPS) in the adult: a consensus approach from the Trans-Atlantic RPS Working Group. Ann Surg Oncol 23(11):3531–3540
18. Trans-AtlanticRetroperitoneal Sarcoma Working Group (TARPSWG) (2018) Management of metastatic retroperitoneal sarcoma: a consensus approach from the Trans-Atlantic Retroperitoneal Sarcoma Working Group (TARPSWG). Ann Oncol 29(4):857–871
19. Gronchi A, Miceli R, Shurell E et al (2013) Outcome prediction in primary resected retroperitoneal soft tissue sarcoma: histology-specific overall survival and disease-free survival nomograms built on major sarcoma center data sets. J Clin Oncol 31(13):1649–1655

20. Raut CP, Miceli R, Strauss DC et al (2016) External validation of a multi-institutional retroperitoneal sarcoma nomogram. Cancer 122(9):1417–1424

21. Gronchi A, Strauss DC, Miceli R et al (2016) Variability in patterns of recurrence after resection of primary retroperitoneal sarcoma (RPS): a report on 1007 patients from the Multi-institutional Collaborative RPS Working Group. Ann Surg 263(5):1002–1009

22. Tan MC, Brennan MF, Kuk D et al (2016) Histology-based classification predicts pattern of recurrence and improves risk stratification in primary retroperitoneal sarcoma. Ann Surg 263(3):593–600

23. Gronchi A, Miceli R, Allard MA et al (2015) Personalizing the approach to retroperitoneal soft tissue sarcoma: histology-specific patterns of failure and postrelapse outcome after primary extended resection. Ann Surg Oncol 22(5):1447–1454

24. Callegaro D, Fiore M, Gronchi A (2015) Personalizing surgical margins in retroperitoneal sarcomas. Expert Rev Anticancer Ther 15(5):553–567

25. MacNeill AJ, Gronchi A, Miceli R et al (2018) Postoperative morbidity after radical resection of primary retroperitoneal sarcoma: a report from the Transatlantic RPS Working Group. Ann Surg 267(5):959–964

26. Tseng WW, Tsao-Wei DD, Callegaro D et al (2018) Pancreaticoduodenectomy in the surgical management of primary retroperitoneal sarcoma. Eur J Surg Oncol 44(6):810–815

27. MacNeill AJ, Miceli R, Strauss DC et al (2017) Post-relapse outcomes after primary extended resection of retroperitoneal sarcoma: a report from the Trans-Atlantic RPS Working Group. Cancer 123(11):1971–1978

Printed in September 2018

Printed in the United States
By Bookmasters